Third Edition

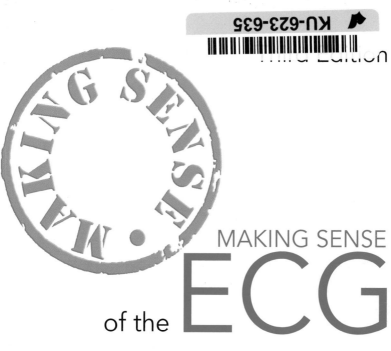

MAKING SENSE

of the ECG

A HANDS-ON GUIDE

Andrew R. Houghton
MA(Oxon) DM FRCP(Lond) FRCP(Glasg)
Consultant Cardiologist
Grantham and District Hospital
Grantham, UK
and
Visiting Fellow, University of Lincoln,
Lincoln, UK

David Gray
DM MPH BMedSci FRCP(Lond) FRIPH
Reader in Medicine and Honorary
Consultant Physician
Department of Cardiovascular Medicine
University Hospital, Queen's Medical Centre,
Nottingham, UK

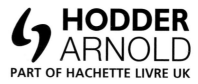

**HODDER
ARNOLD**
PART OF HACHETTE LIVRE UK

First published in Great Britain in 1997 by Arnold
Second edition 2003 by Hodder Arnold
This third edition published in 2008 by
Hodder Arnold, an imprint of Hodder Education, part of Hachette Livre UK,
338 Euston Road, London NW1 3BH

http://www.hoddereducation.com

Whilst the advice and information in this book are believed to be true and accurate
at the date of going to press, neither the author[s] nor the publisher can accept any
legal responsibility or liability for any errors or omissions that may be made. In particular (but without limiting the generality of the preceding disclaimer) every effort
has been made to check drug dosages; however it is still possible that errors have
been missed. Furthermore, dosage schedules are constantly being revised and new
side-effects recognized. For these reasons the reader is strongly urged to consult
the drug companies' printed instructions before administering any of the drugs
recommended in this book.

British Library Cataloguing in Publication Data
A catalogue record for this book is available from the British Library

Library of Congress Cataloging-in-Publication Data
A catalog record for this book is available from the Library of Congress

ISBN   978 0 340 946 886
ISBN [ISE] 978 0 340 946 923 (International Students' Edition, restricted territorial
availability)

1 2 3 4 5 6 7 8 9 10

Commissioning Editor: Sara Purdy
Project Editor: Jane Tod
Production Controller: Andre Sim
Cover Designer: Helen Townson
Indexer: Lisa Footitt

Typeset in 11.5/13 Chaparral by Charon Tec Ltd (A Macmillan Company),
Chennai, India
www.charontec.com
Printed and bound in India

What do you think about this book? Or any other Hodder Arnold title?
Please visit our website: www.hoddereducation.com

To Kathryn and Caroline

Contents

Where to find the ECGs viii
Where to find the medical conditions xiii
Preface to the third edition xvii
Acknowledgements xix

1 PQRST: Where the waves come from 1
2 Heart rate 19
3 Rhythm 28
4 The axis 80
5 The P wave 100
6 The PR interval 112
7 The Q wave 127
8 The QRS complex 135
9 The ST segment 158
10 The T wave 186
11 The QT interval 201
12 The U wave 213
13 Artefacts on the ECG 217
14 Pacemakers and implantable cardioverter defibrillators 222
15 Ambulatory ECG recording 232
16 Exercise ECG testing 239
17 Cardiopulmonary resuscitation 250
18 A history of the ECG 268

Useful websites and further reading 273
Help with the next edition 275

Index 277

Where to find the ECGs

Accelerated idioventricular rhythm Fig. 3.19 — 56

Anterior myocardial infarction Figs 1.10, 7.4, 9.5, 10.3 — 8, 130, 165, 190

Asystole Fig. 17.4 — 260

Atrial ectopics Fig. 3.24 — 61

Atrial fibrillation Figs 3.13, 5.2 — 43, 102

Atrial flutter (3:1 AV block) Fig. 3.11 — 40

Atrial tachycardia Fig. 3.9 — 38

AV block, 2:1 Fig. 6.10 — 123

AV block, first-degree Fig. 6.7 — 119

AV block, Mobitz type I Fig. 6.8 — 121

AV block, Mobitz type II Fig. 6.9 — 122

AV block, third-degree Figs 3.31, 6.11 — 73, 124

AV dissociation Fig. 3.32 — 74

AV junctional ectopics Fig. 3.25 — 62

AV junctional escape rhythm Fig. 3.22 — 60

AV junctional tachycardia Figs 5.4, 5.7 — 104, 107

AV nodal re-entry tachycardia Fig. 3.17 — 50

AV re-entry tachycardia (WPW syndrome) Fig. 3.16 — 49

Bifascicular block Fig. 4.17 — 94

Bigeminy Fig. 3.27	63
Brugada's syndrome Fig. 9.13	176
Bundle branch block, incomplete left Fig. 8.17	154
Bundle branch block, incomplete right Fig. 8.18	155
Bundle branch block, left Fig. 8.11	149
Bundle branch block, right Fig. 8.15	151
Capture beats Fig. 3.35	77
Carotid sinus massage Fig. 3.12	41
Complete AV block Figs 3.31, 6.11	73, 124
Delta wave (WPW syndrome) Figs 6.4, 6.5	115, 116
Dextrocardia Fig. 8.5	143
Digoxin effect Fig. 9.15	181
Digoxin toxicity Fig. 10.8	198
Dual-chamber sequential pacing Fig. 14.2	228
Ectopic beats, atrial Fig. 3.24	61
Ectopic beats, AV junctional Fig. 3.25	62
Ectopic beats, bigeminy Fig. 3.27	63
Ectopic beats, ventricular Figs 3.26, 3.28, 8.16	63, 69, 153
Electrical alternans Fig. 8.7	145
Electrode misplacement Fig. 13.1	218
Electromechanical dissociation Fig. 17.5	260
Exercise test (coronary artery disease) Fig. 16.3	245
First-degree AV block Fig. 6.7	119
Fusion beats Fig. 3.34	76
High take-off Fig. 9.12	174
Hypercalcaemia Fig. 11.2	205
Hyperkalaemia Fig. 10.2	188
Hypertrophy, left ventricular Figs 7.6, 8.2	133, 138
Hypertrophy, left ventricular with strain Fig. 9.16	183
Hypertrophy, right ventricular with strain Fig. 8.3	140

Hypocalcaemia Fig. 11.3	208
Hypokalaemia Figs 10.4, 12.2	191, 215
Hypothermia 9.17	184
Incomplete left bundle branch block Fig. 8.17	154
Incomplete right bundle branch block Fig 8.18	155
Incorrect calibration Fig. 13.3	219
Incorrect paper speed Fig. 13.4	220
Inferior myocardial infarction Figs 1.9, 7.5, 9.6	8, 131, 166
J point Fig. 16.2	244
Junctional escape beat Fig. 3.6	35
Lateral myocardial infarction Figs 1.10, 9.4	8, 164
Left axis deviation Fig. 4.16	93
Left bundle branch block Fig. 8.11	149
Left bundle branch block, incomplete Fig. 8.17	154
Left ventricular aneurysm Fig. 9.9	169
Left ventricular hypertrophy Figs 7.6, 8.2	133, 138
Left ventricular hypertrophy with strain Fig. 9.16	183
Long QT interval Fig. 11.3	208
Lown – Ganong – Levine syndrome Fig. 6.6	117
Mobitz type I AV block Fig. 6.8	121
Mobitz type II AV block Fig. 6.9	122
Myocardial infarction, anterior Figs 7.4, 9.5, 10.3	130, 165, 190
Myocardial infarction, inferior Figs 1.9, 7.5, 9.6	8, 131, 166
Myocardial infarction, lateral Figs 1.10, 9.4	8, 164
Myocardial infarction, posterior Fig. 8.4	141
Myocardial infarction, Q wave Fig. 10.7	196
Myocardial infarction, right ventricular Fig. 9.8	167
Myocardial ischaemia Figs 9.14, 10.6, 16.3	178, 195, 245
Normal 12-lead ECG Figs 8.1, 10.1	135, 186
Normal T wave inversion Fig. 10.5	193

P mitrale Fig. 5.9	110
P pulmonale Fig. 5.8	108
Pacing – dual-chamber sequential Fig. 14.2	228
Pacing – ventricular Fig. 14.1	228
Pericardial effusion Figs 8.6, 8.7	144, 145
Pericarditis Fig. 9.11	172
Posterior myocardial infarction Fig. 8.4	141
Prinzmetal's angina Fig. 9.10	171
Q wave myocardial infarction Fig. 10.7	196
Q wave, normal Fig. 7.3	129
QT interval, long Fig. 11.3	208
QT interval, short Fig. 11.2	205
Right axis deviation Fig. 4.19	97
Right bundle branch block Fig. 8.15	151
Right bundle branch block, incomplete Fig. 8.18	155
Right ventricular hypertrophy with strain Fig. 8.3	140
Right ventricular myocardial infarction Fig. 9.8	167
Short QT interval Fig. 11.2	205
Signal-averaged ECG Fig. 13.5	221
Sinoatrial block Figs 3.7	36
Sinus arrest Figs 3.6, 5.3	35, 103
Sinus arrhythmia Fig. 3.5	34
Sinus bradycardia Fig. 3.3	31
Sinus rhythm Figs 3.1, 3.2, 5.1	28, 30, 101
Sinus tachycardia Figs 3.4, 5.5	32, 104
T wave inversion (normal) Fig. 10.5	193
Tachycardia, AV junctional Figs 5.4, 5.7	104, 107
Tachycardia, sinus Figs 3.4, 5.5	32, 104
Tachycardia, ventricular Figs 3.18, 3.33, 3.34, 3.35, 17.3	53, 76, 76, 77, 259
Tense patient Fig. 1.1	2

Third-degree AV block Figs 3.31, 6.11	73, 124
Torsades de pointes Fig. 3.20	56
Trifascicular block Fig. 4.18	95
U wave Figs 12.1, 12.2	213, 215
Vasospastic angina Fig. 9.10	171
Ventricular ectopics Figs 3.26, 3.28, 8.16	63, 69, 153
Ventricular escape rhythm Fig. 3.23	60
Ventricular fibrillation Figs 3.18, 17.2	53, 259
Ventricular pacing Fig. 14.1	228
Ventricular tachycardia Figs 3.18, 3.33, 3.34, 3.35, 17.3	53, 76, 76, 77, 259
Wolff–Parkinson–White syndrome Figs 6.4, 6.5	115, 116

Where to find the medical conditions

Abnormal atrial depolarization	106
Accelerated idioventricular rhythm	56
Anterolateral myocardial infarction	98
Asystole	259
Atrial enlargement, left	109
Atrial enlargement, right	107–8
Atrial fibrillation	42
Atrial flutter	39
Atrial tachycardia	37
AV block, 2:1	122
AV block, first-degree	118
AV block, Mobitz type I	119
AV block, Mobitz type II	121
AV block, third-degree	123
AV dissociation	125
AV junctional rhythms	59
AV re-entry tachycardia	47
Bradycardia	21
Brugada syndrome	176
Bundle branch block	147
Complete heart block	123

Conduction disturbances	58
Congenital short QT syndromes	204
Dextrocardia	142
Digoxin	180
Digoxin toxicity	182
Ectopic beats	61
Electromechanical dissociation	260
Escape rhythms	59
Fascicular block	155
First-degree AV block	118
Hemiblock, left anterior	92
Hemiblock, left posterior	98
High take-off	174
Hypercalcaemia	205
Hyperkalaemia	187
Hyperthyroidism	192
Hypertrophy, left ventricular	136
Hypertrophy, right ventricular	139
Hypocalcaemia	208
Hypokalaemia	191
Hypothermia	183
Hypothyroidism	192
Incomplete bundle branch block	154
Inferior myocardial infarction	96
Jervell and Lange-Nielsen syndrome	211
Left anterior hemiblock	92
Left atrial enlargement	109
Left anterior hemiblock	92
Left posterior hemiblock	98
Left ventricular aneurysm	169

Left ventricular hypertrophy	133
Long QT syndrome	211
Lown–Ganong–Levine syndrome	117
Mobitz type I AV block	120
Mobitz type II AV block	121
Myocardial infarction	196
Myocardial infarction, anterolateral	164
Myocardial infarction, inferior	164
Myocardial infarction, posterior	139
Myocardial infarction, right ventricular	165, 167
Myocardial ischaemia	177
Myocarditis	210
Non-ST segment elevation acute coronary syndrome	160
Pacemakers and surgery	229
Pericardial effusion	144
Pericarditis	172
Posterior myocardial infarction	139
Prinzmetal's angina	170
Pulseless ventricular tachycardia	259
Right atrial enlargement	107–8
Right ventricular hypertrophy	139
Right ventricular myocardial infarction	165, 167
Romano–Ward syndrome	211
Sick sinus syndrome	35
Sinus arrhythmia	34
Sinus bradycardia	31
Sinus rhythm	29
Sinus tachycardia	32
ST segment elevation acute coronary syndrome	159
Surgery and pacemakers	229

Tachycardia	24
Third-degree AV block	123
Torsades de pointes	56
Unstable angina	179
Vasospastic angina	170
Ventricular fibrillation	57
Ventricular hypertrophy	136
Ventricular hypertrophy with strain	182
Ventricular rhythms	53
Ventricular tachycardia	53
Ventricular tachycardia, pulseless	259
Wolff–Parkinson–White syndrome	96

Preface to the third edition

The first question that occurs to any authors contemplating a new edition of a textbook is 'What's new?' Since our second edition, published in 2003, there have been a lot of developments.

First and foremost, the Resuscitation Council (UK) has completely revised its guidelines and this had necessitated a complete re-write of the chapter on cardiopulmonary resuscitation.

There have been significant developments in the field of arrhythmias, and we have added new material on conditions such as Brugada syndrome and the long QT syndrome, together with the latest National Institute for Health and Clinical Excellence (NICE) guidance on atrial fibrillation and updated material on interventions such as pulmonary vein isolation.

The diagnosis and management of acute coronary syndromes also continues to evolve, and the sections on ischaemic heart disease have been updated accordingly.

We have also taken the opportunity to review and upgrade the entire text, improving the clarity of the information wherever possible and also adding new material on, for example, the history of the ECG. Last, but by no means least, we have replaced many of the ECGs with clearer and better examples.

Once again, we are grateful to everyone who has taken the time to comment on the text and to provide us with ECGs from their collections. Finally, we would like to thank all the staff at Hodder Arnold who have contributed to the success of *Making Sense of the ECG: A hands-on guide*.

Andrew R Houghton
David Gray
2008

Acknowledgements

We would like to thank everyone who gave us suggestions and constructive criticism while we prepared the first, second and third editions of *Making Sense of the ECG*. We are particularly grateful to the following for their invaluable comments on the text and for allowing us to use ECGs from their collections:

Mookhter Ajij
Khin Maung Aye
Stephanie Baker
Michael Bamber
Muneer Ahmad Bhat
Gabriella Captur
Andrea Charman
Matthew Donnelly
Ian Ferrer
Lawrence Green
Mahesh Harishchandra
Michael Holmes
Safiy Karim
Dave Kendall
Daniel Law
Diane Lunn
Iain Lyburn
Sonia Lyburn

Martin Melville
Cara Mercer
Yuji Murakawa
Francis Murgatroyd
V B S Naidu
Vicky Nelmes
Claire Poole
George B Pradhān
Jane Robinson
Catherine Scott
Penelope R Sensky
Neville Smith
Gary Spiers
Andrew Stein
Robin Touquet
Upul Wijayawardhana
Bernadette Williamson

We are grateful to the *New England Journal of Medicine* for permission to adapt material from the journal for Chapter 16, and

ACKNOWLEDGEMENTS

to the Resuscitation Council (UK) for permission to reproduce the adult Advanced Life Support algorithm in Chapter 17.

Finally, we would also like to express our gratitude to everyone at Hodder Arnold for their guidance and support.

1 PQRST: Where the waves come from

The electrocardiogram (ECG) is one of the most widely used and useful investigations in contemporary medicine. It is essential for the identification of disorders of the cardiac rhythm, extremely useful for the diagnosis of abnormalities of the heart (such as myocardial infarction), and a helpful clue to the presence of generalized disorders that affect the rest of the body too (such as electrolyte disturbances).

Each chapter in this book considers a specific feature of the ECG in turn. We begin, however, with an overview of the ECG in which we explain the following points:

- What does the ECG actually record?
- How does the ECG 'look' at the heart?
- Where do the waves come from?
- How do I record an ECG?

We recommend you take some time to read through this chapter before trying to interpret ECG abnormalities.

● What does the ECG actually record?

ECG machines record the electrical activity of the heart. They also pick up the activity of other muscles, such as skeletal muscle, but are designed to filter this out as much as possible.

Encouraging patients to relax during an ECG recording helps to obtain a clear trace (Fig. 1.1).

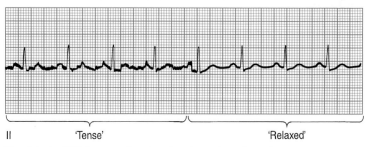

II   'Tense'   'Relaxed'

Fig. 1.1 An ECG from a relaxed patient is much easier to interpret

Key points: • electrical interference (irregular baseline) when patient is tense
             • clearer recording when patient relaxes

By convention, the main waves on the ECG are given the names P, Q, R, S, T and U (Fig. 1.2). Each wave represents depolarization ('electrical discharging') or repolarization ('electrical recharging') of a certain region of the heart – this is discussed in more detail in the rest of this chapter.

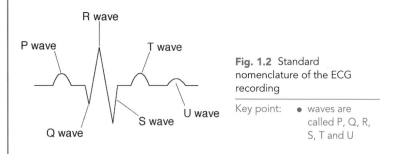

R wave

P wave   T wave

                                    U wave

          Q wave   S wave

Fig. 1.2 Standard nomenclature of the ECG recording

Key point: • waves are called P, Q, R, S, T and U

The voltage changes detected by ECG machines are very small, being of the order of millivolts. The size of each wave corresponds to the amount of voltage generated by the event that created it: the greater the voltage, the larger the wave (Fig. 1.3).

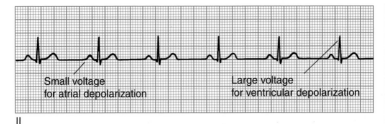

II

Fig. 1.3 The size of a wave reflects the voltage that caused it

Key points:
- P waves are small (atrial depolarization generates little voltage)
- QRS complexes are larger (ventricular depolarization generates a higher voltage)

The ECG also allows you to calculate how long an event lasted. The ECG paper moves through the machine at a constant rate of 25 mm/s, so by measuring the width of a P wave, for example, you can calculate the duration of atrial depolarization (Fig. 1.4).

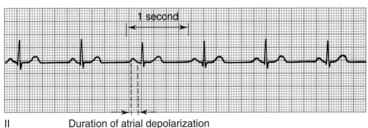

II

Duration of atrial depolarization
= 0.10 seconds

1 large square =   1 small square =
0.2 seconds   0.04 seconds

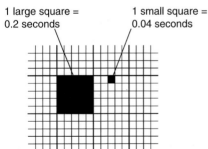

Fig. 1.4 The width of a wave reflects an event's duration

Key points:
- the P waves are 2.5 mm wide
- atrial depolarization therefore took 0.10 s

● How does the ECG 'look' at the heart?

To make sense of the ECG, one of the most important concepts to understand is that of the 'lead'. This is a term you will often see, and it does *not* refer to the wires that connect the patient to the ECG machine (which we will always refer to as 'electrodes' to avoid confusion).

In short, 'leads' are different *viewpoints* of the heart's electrical activity. An ECG machine uses the information it collects via its four limb and six chest electrodes to compile a comprehensive picture of the electrical activity in the heart as observed from 12 different viewpoints, and this set of 12 views or leads gives the 12-lead ECG its name.

Each lead is given a name (I, II, III, aVR, aVL, aVF, V_1, V_2, V_3, V_4, V_5 and V_6) and its position on a 12-lead ECG is usually standardized to make pattern recognition easier.

● ECG lead nomenclature

There are several ways of categorizing the 12 ECG leads. They are often referred to as limb leads (I, II, III, aVR, aVL, aVF) and chest leads (V_1, V_2, V_3, V_4, V_5, V_6). They can also be divided into bipolar leads (I, II, III) or unipolar leads (aVR, aVL, aVF, V_1, V_2, V_3, V_4, V_5, V_6).

Bipolar leads are generated by measuring the voltage between two electrodes, for example, lead I measures the voltage between the left arm electrode and the right arm electrode. Unipolar leads measure the voltage between a single positive electrode and a 'central' point of reference generated from the other electrodes, for example, lead aVR uses the right arm electrode as the positive terminal.

So what viewpoint does each lead have of the heart? Information from the four limb electrodes is used by the ECG machine to create the six limb leads (I, II, III, aVR, aVL and aVF). Each limb lead 'looks' at the heart from the side (the coronal plane), and the angle at which it looks at the heart in this plane depends on the lead in question (Fig. 1.5). Thus, lead aVR looks at the heart from the approximate viewpoint of the patient's right shoulder, whereas lead aVL looks from the left shoulder and lead aVF looks directly upward from the feet.

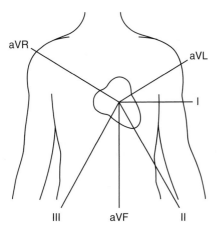

Fig. 1.5 The viewpoint each limb lead has of the heart

Key points:
- each limb lead looks at the heart in the coronal plane
- each limb lead looks at the heart from a different angle

The six chest leads (V_1–V_6) look at the heart in a horizontal plane from the front and around the side of the chest (Fig. 1.6).

The region of myocardium surveyed by each lead therefore varies according to its vantage point – lead aVF has a good 'view' of the inferior surface of the heart, and lead V_3 has a good view of the anterior surface, for example.

Once you know the view each lead has of the heart, you can tell if the electrical impulses in the heart are flowing towards that lead or away from it. This is simple to work out, because electrical current flowing towards a lead produces an upward (positive) deflection on the ECG, whereas current flowing away causes a downward (negative) deflection (Fig. 1.7).

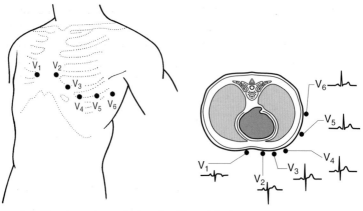

Fig. 1.6 The viewpoint each chest lead has of the heart

Key points:
- each chest lead looks at the heart in the transverse plane
- each chest lead looks at the heart from a different angle

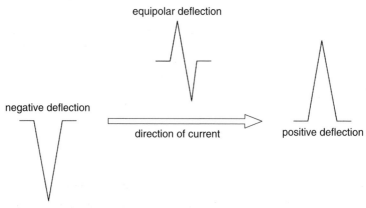

Fig. 1.7 The direction of an ECG deflection depends on the direction of the current

Key points:
- flow towards a lead produces a positive deflection
- flow away from a lead produces a negative deflection
- flow past a lead produces a positive then a negative (equipolar) deflection

We will discuss the origin of each wave shortly, but just as an example consider the P wave, which represents atrial depolarization. The P wave is positive in lead II because atrial depolarization flows towards that lead, but it is negative in lead aVR because this lead looks at the atria from the opposite direction (Fig. 1.8).

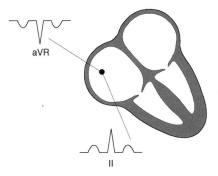

Fig. 1.8 The orientation of the P wave depends on the lead

Key points:
- P waves are normally upright in lead II
- P waves are normally inverted in lead aVR

In addition to working out the direction of flow of electrical current, knowing the viewpoint of each lead allows you to determine which regions of the heart are affected by, for example, a myocardial infarction. Infarction of the inferior surface will produce changes in the leads looking at that region, namely leads II, III and aVF (Fig. 1.9). An anterior infarction produces changes mainly in leads V_1–V_4 (Fig. 1.10).

● Why are there 12 ECG leads?

Twelve leads simply provide a number of different views of the heart that are manageable (too many leads would take too long to interpret) and yet provide a comprehensive picture of the heart's electrical activity (too few leads might 'overlook' important regions). For research purposes, where a more detailed picture of the heart is needed, over 100 leads are often used.

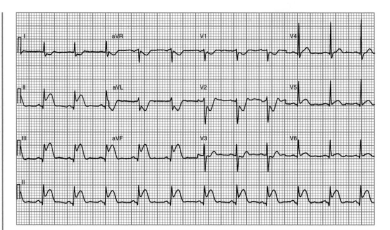

Fig. 1.9 An inferior myocardial infarction produces changes in the inferior leads

Key points:
- leads II, III and aVF look at the inferior surface of the heart
- ST segment elevation is present in these leads (acute inferior myocardial infarction)
- there are also reciprocal changes in leads V_1–V_3, I and aVL

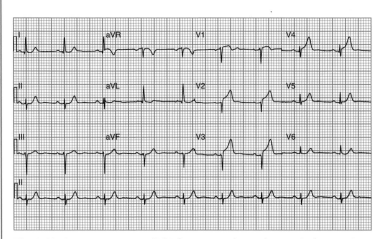

Fig. 1.10 An anterior myocardial infarction produces changes in the anterior leads

Key points:
- leads V_1–V_4 look at the anterior surface of the heart
- ST segment elevation is present in these leads, with Q waves in V_1–V_3 (anterior myocardial infarction after 24 h)

● Where do the waves come from?

In the normal heart, each beat begins with the discharge ('depolarization') of the sinoatrial (SA) node, high up in the right atrium. This is a spontaneous event, occurring 60–100 times every minute.

Depolarization of the SA node does not cause any noticeable wave on the standard ECG (although it can be seen on specialized intracardiac recordings). The first detectable wave appears when the impulse spreads from the SA node to depolarize the atria (Fig. 1.11). This produces the **P wave**.

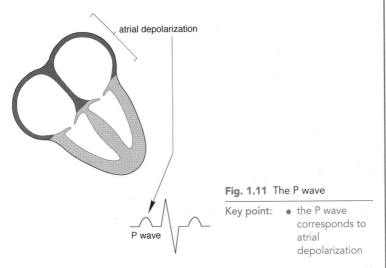

atrial depolarization

P wave

Fig. 1.11 The P wave

Key point: ● the P wave corresponds to atrial depolarization

The atria contain relatively little muscle, so the voltage generated by atrial depolarization is relatively small. From the viewpoint of most leads, the electricity appears to flow *towards* them and so the P wave will be a positive (upward) deflection. The exception is lead aVR, where the electricity appears to flow *away*, and so the P wave is negative in that lead (see Fig. 1.8).

After flowing through the atria, the electrical impulse reaches the atrioventricular (AV) node, located low in the right atrium. The AV node is normally the only route by which an electrical impulse can reach the ventricles, the rest of the atrial myocardium being separated from the ventricles by a non-conducting ring of fibrous tissue.

Activation of the AV node does not produce an obvious wave on the ECG, but it does contribute to the time interval between the P wave and the subsequent Q or R wave. It does this by delaying conduction, and in doing so acts as a safety mechanism, preventing rapid atrial impulses (for instance during atrial flutter or fibrillation) from spreading to the ventricles at the same rate.

The time taken for the depolarization wave to pass from its origin in the SA node, across the atria, and through the AV node into ventricular muscle is called the **PR interval**. This is measured from the beginning of the P wave to the beginning of the R wave, and is normally between 0.12 s and 0.20 s, or three to five small squares on the ECG paper (Fig. 1.12).

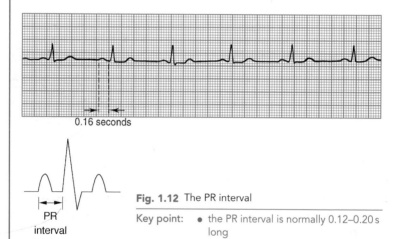

0.16 seconds

PR interval

Fig. 1.12 The PR interval

Key point: • the PR interval is normally 0.12–0.20 s long

Once the impulse has traversed the AV node, it enters the bundle of His, a specialized conducting pathway that passes into the interventricular septum and divides into the left and right bundle branches (Fig. 1.13).

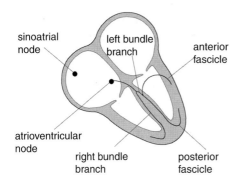

sinoatrial node

left bundle branch

anterior fascicle

atrioventricular node

right bundle branch

posterior fascicle

Fig. 1.13 The right and left bundle branches

Key point: • the bundle of His divides into the right and left bundle branches in the inter-ventricular septum

Current normally flows between the bundle branches in the interventricular septum, from left to right, and this is respon-sible for the first deflection of the **QRS complex**. Whether this is a downward deflection or an upward deflection depends on which side of the septum a lead is 'looking' from (Fig. 1.14).

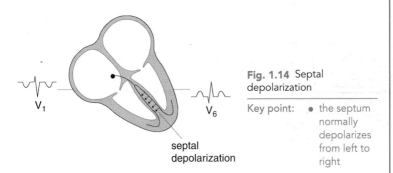

V_1

V_6

septal depolarization

Fig. 1.14 Septal depolarization

Key point: • the septum normally depolarizes from left to right

By convention, if the first deflection of the QRS complex is downward, it is called a **Q wave**. The first upward deflection is called an **R wave**, whether or not it follows a Q wave. A down-ward deflection after an R wave is called an **S wave**. Hence, a variety of complexes is possible (Fig. 1.15).

The right bundle branch conducts the wave of depolarization to the right ventricle, whereas the left bundle branch divides into anterior and posterior fascicles that conduct the wave to the left ventricle (Fig. 1.16). The conducting pathways end by dividing into Purkinje fibres that distribute the wave of depolarization

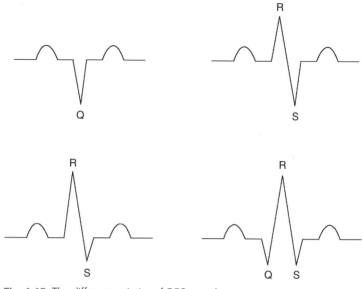

Fig. 1.15 The different varieties of QRS complex

Key points:
- the first downward deflection is a Q wave
- the first upward deflection is an R wave
- a downward deflection after an R wave is an S wave

rapidly throughout both ventricles. The depolarization of the ventricles, represented by the QRS complex, is normally complete within 0.12 s (Fig. 1.17). QRS complexes are 'positive' or 'negative', depending on whether the R wave or the S wave is bigger (Fig. 1.18). This, in turn, will depend on the view each lead has of the heart.

The left ventricle contains considerably more myocardium than the right, and so the voltage generated by its depolarization will tend to dominate the shape of the QRS complex.

Leads that look at the heart from the right will see a relatively small amount of voltage moving towards them as the right ventricle depolarizes, and a larger amount moving away with depolarization of the left ventricle. The QRS complex will therefore be dominated by an S wave, and be negative. Conversely, leads looking at the heart from the left will see a relatively large voltage

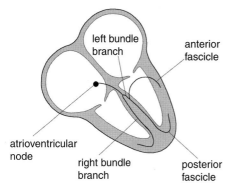

Fig. 1.16 Divisions of the left bundle branch

Key point: • the left bundle branch divides into anterior and posterior fascicles

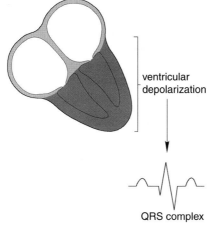

ventricular depolarization

Fig. 1.17 The QRS complex

Key point: • the QRS complex corresponds to ventricular depolarization

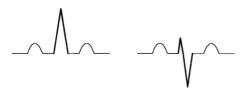

positive   negative   equipolar

Fig. 1.18 Polarity of the QRS complexes

Key points: • a dominant R wave means a positive QRS complex
• a dominant S wave means a negative QRS complex
• equal R and S waves mean an equipolar QRS complex

moving towards them, and a smaller voltage moving away, giving rise to a large R wave and only a small S wave (Fig. 1.19). Therefore, there is a gradual transition across the chest leads, from a predominantly negative QRS complex to a predominantly positive one (Fig. 1.20).

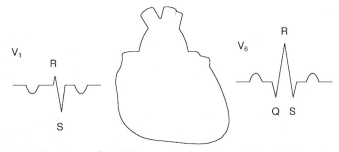

Fig. 1.19 The shape of the QRS complex depends on the lead's viewpoint

Key points:
- right-sided leads have negative QRS complexes
- left-sided leads have positive QRS complexes

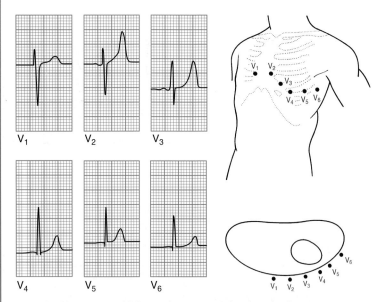

Fig. 1.20 Transition in QRS complexes across the chest leads

Key points:
- QRS complexes are normally negative in leads V_1 and V_2
- QRS complexes are normally positive in leads V_5 and V_6

The **ST segment** is the transient period in which no more electrical current can be passed through the myocardium. It is measured from the end of the S wave to the beginning of the T wave (Fig. 1.21). The ST segment is of particular interest in the diagnosis of myocardial infarction and ischaemia (see Chapter 9).

The **T wave** represents repolarization ('recharging') of the ventricular myocardium to its resting electrical state. The **QT interval** measures the total time for activation of the ventricles and recovery to the normal resting state (Fig. 1.22).

The origin of the **U wave** is uncertain, but it may represent repolarization of the interventricular septum or slow repolarization of the ventricles. U waves can be difficult to identify but, when present, they are most clearly seen in the anterior chest leads V_2–V_4 (Fig. 1.23).

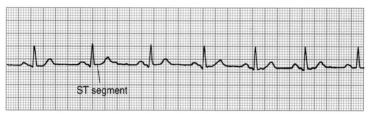

Fig. 1.21 The ST segment

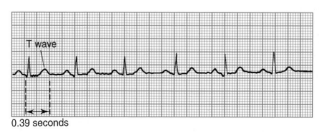

0.39 seconds

Fig. 1.22 The T wave and QT interval

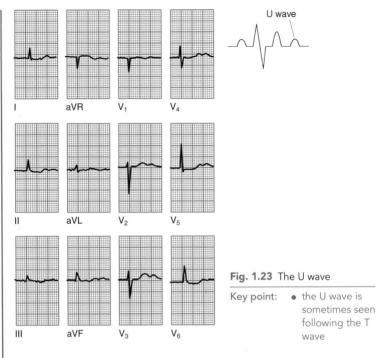

U wave

Fig. 1.23 The U wave

Key point: • the U wave is sometimes seen following the T wave

You need to be familiar with the most important electrical events that make up the cardiac cycle. These are summarized at the end of the chapter.

● How do I record an ECG?

Ensure that you know how to operate the ECG machine before attempting to record an ECG. An incorrect recording can lead to incorrect diagnoses, wasted investigations and potentially disastrous unnecessary treatment.

To record a clear, noise-free ECG, begin by asking the patient to lie down and relax to reduce electrical interference from skeletal muscle. Before attaching the electrodes, prepare the skin underneath with a spirit wipe and remove excess hair to ensure good electrical contact.

Attach the limb and chest electrodes in their correct positions. The limb electrodes are usually labelled and/or colour coded according to which arm or leg they need to be attached. Most modern machines have six chest electrodes, which will also be labelled or colour coded, and these need to be positioned as shown in Figure 1.24. Older machines may have only one chest electrode, which needs to be repositioned to record each of the six chest leads.

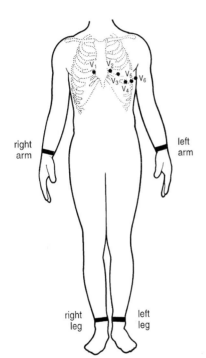

right arm

left arm

right leg

left leg

Fig. 1.24 Electrode positions on the limbs and chest

Key point: • always ensure the electrodes are correctly positioned

When recording the ECG, always check that the machine is properly calibrated so that:

- the paper speed is correct (25 mm/s is standard)
- the calibration mark has been made, such that 10 mm = 1 mV, so that wave height can readily be converted into a more meaningful voltage.

The recognition of artefacts on the ECG is discussed in Chapter 13.

Summary

The waves and intervals of the ECG correspond to the following events:

ECG event	Cardiac event
P wave	Atrial depolarization
PR interval	Start of atrial depolarization to start of ventricular depolarization
QRS complex	Ventricular depolarization
ST segment	Pause in ventricular electrical activity before repolarization
T wave	Ventricular repolarization
QT interval	Total time taken by ventricular depolarization and repolarization
U wave	Uncertain – possibly: • interventricular septal repolarization • slow ventricular repolarization

Note. Depolarizations of the SA and AV nodes are important events but do not *in themselves* produce a detectable wave on the standard ECG.

2 Heart rate

Measurement of the heart rate and the identification of the cardiac rhythm go hand in hand, as many abnormalities of heart rate result from arrhythmias. Chapter 3 discusses in detail how to identify the cardiac rhythm. To begin with, however, we will simply describe ways to measure the heart rate and the abnormalities that can affect it.

When we talk of measuring the heart rate, we usually mean the *ventricular* rate, which corresponds to the patient's pulse. Depolarization of the ventricles produces the QRS complex on the ECG, and so it is the rate of QRS complexes that needs to be measured to determine the heart rate.

Measurement of the heart rate is simple and can be done in several ways. However, before you try to measure anything, check that the ECG has been recorded at the standard UK and US paper speed of 25 mm/s. If so, then all you have to remember is that a 1-min ECG tracing covers **300 large squares**. If the patient's rhythm is regular, all you have to do is count the number of large squares between two consecutive QRS complexes, and divide it into 300.

For example, in Figure 2.1 there are 5 large squares between each QRS complex. Therefore:

$$\text{Heart rate} = \frac{300}{5} = 60/\text{min}$$

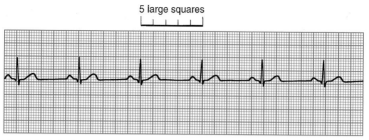

Fig. 2.1 Calculating heart rate when the rhythm is regular

Key points:
- 1 QRS complex every 5 large squares
- 300 large squares correspond to 1 min

This method does not work so well when the rhythm is irregular, as the number of large squares between each QRS complex varies from beat to beat. So, instead, count the number of QRS complexes in 30 large squares (Fig. 2.2). This is the number of QRS complexes in 6 s. To work out the rate/min, simply multiply by 10:

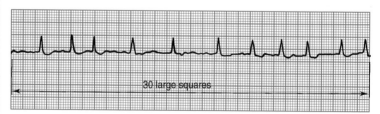

Fig. 2.2 Calculating heart rate when the rhythm is irregular

Key points:
- 30 large squares contain 11 QRS complexes
- 30 large squares correspond to 6 s

Number of QRS complexes in 30 squares = 11

Therefore, number of QRS complexes in 6 s = 11

Therefore, number of QRS complexes/min = 11 × 10 = 110

An ECG ruler can be helpful, but follow the instructions on it carefully. Some ECG machines will calculate heart rate and print it on the ECG, but always check machine-derived values, as machines do occasionally make errors!

Whichever method you use, remember it can also be used to measure the atrial or P wave rate as well as the ventricular or QRS rate. Normally, every P wave is followed by a QRS complex and so the atrial and ventricular rates are the same. However, the rates can be different if, for example, some or all of the P waves are prevented from activating the ventricles (Fig. 2.3). Situations where this may happen are described in later chapters.

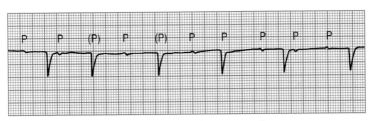

Fig. 2.3 The P wave rate can differ from the QRS complex rate

Key points: ● P wave (atrial) rate is 105/min
            ● QRS complex (ventricular) rate is 60/min

Once you have measured the heart rate, you need to decide whether it is normal or abnormal. As a general rule, a regular heart rhythm with a rate between 60 and 100 beats/min is normal. If the rate is below 60 beats/min, the patient is said to be **bradycardic**. With a heart rate above 100 beats/min, the patient is **tachycardic**. Therefore, the two questions you need to ask about heart rate are:

● Is the heart rate below 60 beats/min?
● Is the heart rate above 100 beats/min?

If the answer to either question is 'yes', turn to the appropriate half of this chapter to find out what to do next. If not, turn to Chapter 3 to identify the cardiac rhythm.

● Is the heart rate below 60 beats/min?

Bradycardia is arbitrarily defined as a heart rate below 60 beats/min. Identification of the cardiac rhythm and any conduction disturbances is essential, and this is discussed in Chapter 3.

Problems to consider in the bradycardic patient are:

- sinus bradycardia
- sick sinus syndrome
- second-degree and third-degree atrioventricular (AV) block
- 'escape' rhythms
- AV junctional escape rhythm
- ventricular escape rhythms
- asystole.

Sinus bradycardia (p. 31) can be normal, for example in athletes during sleep, but in others it may indicate an underlying problem. The differential diagnosis and treatment are discussed in Chapter 3.

Sick sinus syndrome (p. 35) is the coexistence of sinus bradycardia with episodes of sinus arrest and sinoatrial block. Patients may also have episodes of paroxysmal tachycardia, giving rise to the tachy-brady syndrome.

In **second-degree AV block** (p. 58) some atrial impulses fail to be conducted to the ventricles, and this can lead to bradycardia. In **third-degree AV block**, no atrial impulses can reach the ventricles; in response, the ventricles usually develop an 'escape' rhythm (see below). It is important to remember that AV block can coexist with *any* atrial rhythm.

Escape rhythms (p. 59 are a form of 'safety net' to maintain a heart beat if the normal mechanism of impulse generation fails or is blocked. They may also appear during episodes of severe sinus bradycardia. The distinction between AV junctional and ventricular escape rhythms is discussed in Chapter 3.

Asystole (p. 259) implies the absence of ventricular activity, and so the heart rate is zero. Asystole is a medical emergency and requires immediate diagnosis and treatment if the patient is to have any chance of survival. A management algorithm is given in Figure 17.1 (p. 256).

Do not forget that arrhythmias that are usually associated with normal or fast heart rates may be slowed by certain drugs, resulting in bradycardia. For example, patients with atrial fibrillation (which if untreated may cause a *tachycardia*) can develop a *bradycardia* when commenced on anti-arrhythmic drugs. Table 2.1 lists drugs that commonly slow the heart rate (**negatively chronotropic**). A thorough review of all the patient's current and recent medications is therefore essential.

Table 2.1 Negatively chronotropic drugs

- Beta blockers (do not forget eye drops)
- Some calcium antagonists, e.g. verapamil, diltiazem
- Digoxin
- Adenosine

DRUG POINT

A complete drug history is essential in any patient with an abnormal ECG.

The first step in managing a bradycardia is to assess the urgency of the situation. Ask the patient about symptoms of dizziness, syncope, falls, fatigue, breathlessness, chest pain and palpitations. Perform a thorough examination, looking particularly for evidence of haemodynamic disturbance such as hypotension, cardiac failure and poor peripheral perfusion.

Use the history, examination and investigations (e.g. plasma electrolytes, thyroid function tests) to identify any underlying cause, and correct it where possible. When bradycardia is severe and symptomatic, urgent treatment is required:

- atropine 300–600 mcg given slowly intravenously (do not exceed 3 mg in 24 h).

However, if a pacemaker is likely to be needed (see Chapter 14), use atropine only as a short-term measure while arranging for temporary pacing.

Chronic bradycardia may be an indication for a permanent pacemaker, particularly when it is causing symptoms or haemodynamic disturbance. Referral to a cardiologist is recommended.

SEEK HELP

Bradycardias may require pacing, especially if symptomatic. Seek advice from a cardiologist without delay.

● Is the heart rate above 100 beats/min?

Tachycardia is arbitrarily defined as a heart rate above 100 beats/min. When a patient presents with a tachycardia, you must begin by identifying the cardiac rhythm. See Chapter 3 for specific descriptions of how to recognize and manage each rhythm.

Begin the process of identification by checking whether the QRS complexes are:

- narrow (<3 small squares)
- broad (>3 small squares).

Narrow-complex tachycardias always arise from above the ventricles – that is, they are supraventricular in origin. The possibilities are:

- sinus tachycardia
- atrial tachycardia
- atrial flutter
- atrial fibrillation
- AV re-entry tachycardias.

All of these are discussed in detail in Chapter 3.

Broad QRS complexes can occur if normal electrical impulses are conducted abnormally or 'aberrantly' to the ventricles. This delays ventricular activation, widening the QRS complex. Any of the supraventricular tachycardias (SVTs) listed above can also present as a **broad-complex tachycardia** if aberrant conduction is present.

Broad-complex tachycardia should also make you think of ventricular arrhythmias:

- ventricular tachycardia
- accelerated idioventricular rhythm
- torsades de pointes.

Each of these, including aberrant conduction, is discussed in Chapter 3. How to distinguish between ventricular tachycardia and SVT is discussed on page 74.

Ventricular fibrillation (VF) is hard to categorize. The chaotic nature of the underlying ventricular activity can give rise to a variety of ECG appearances, but all have the characteristics of being unpredictable and chaotic. Ventricular fibrillation is a medical emergency and so it is important that you can recognize it immediately; you should read Chapter 17 carefully if you are not confident in doing so.

Management of tachycardia depends on the underlying rhythm, and the treatment of the different arrhythmias is detailed in Chapter 3. The first step, as with managing a bradycardia, is to assess the urgency of the situation.

Clues to the nature of the arrhythmia may be found in the patient's history. Ask the patient about:

- how any palpitations start and stop (sudden or gradual)
- whether there are any situations in which they are more likely to happen (e.g. during exercise, lying quietly in bed)
- how long they last
- whether there are any associated symptoms (dizziness, syncope, falls, fatigue, breathlessness and chest pain).

Also ask the patient to 'tap out' how the palpitations feel – this will give you clues about the rate (fast or slow) and rhythm (regular or irregular).

Also enquire about symptoms of related disorders (e.g. hyperthyroidism) and obtain a list of current medications. Check for any drugs (e.g. salbutamol) that can increase the heart rate (**positively chronotropic**). Do not forget to ask about caffeine intake (coffee, tea and cola drinks).

A thorough examination is always important, looking for evidence of haemodynamic disturbance (hypotension, cardiac failure and poor peripheral perfusion) and coexistent disorders (e.g. thyroid goitre).

Use the history, examination and further investigations (e.g. plasma electrolytes, thyroid function tests) to reach a diagnosis. Ambulatory ECG recording may be helpful if circumstances permit it (see Chapter 15).

In an emergency, every effort must be made to diagnose and correct the rhythm as quickly as possible. If the diagnosis is unclear and the patient needs immediate treatment, most tachycardias will respond to direct current cardioversion. Do not hesitate to seek the urgent advice of a cardiologist if circumstances permit.

ACT QUICKLY

Tachycardia causing haemodynamic disturbance requires urgent diagnosis and treatment.

Summary

To assess the heart rate, ask the following questions.

1. Is the heart rate below 60 beats/min?

If 'yes', consider:

- sinus bradycardia
- sick sinus syndrome
- second-degree and third-degree AV block
- escape rhythms
  - AV junctional escape rhythm
  - ventricular escape rhythms
  - asystole
  - drug-induced condition.

2. Is the heart rate above 100 beats/min?

If 'yes', consider:

- narrow-complex tachycardia
  - sinus tachycardia
  - atrial tachycardia
  - atrial flutter
  - atrial fibrillation
  - AV re-entry tachycardias
- broad-complex tachycardia
  - narrow-complex tachycardia with aberrant conduction
  - ventricular tachycardia
  - accelerated idioventricular rhythm
  - torsades de pointes.

Rhythm **3**

To identify the cardiac rhythm with confidence you need to examine a rhythm strip – a prolonged recording of the ECG from just one lead, usually lead II (Fig. 3.1). Most ECG machines automatically include a rhythm strip at the bottom of a 12-lead ECG. If your machine does not, make sure you have recorded one yourself. The diagnosis of rhythm abnormalities may only become apparent when you examine 12 or more consecutive complexes.

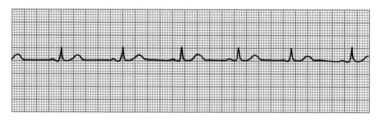

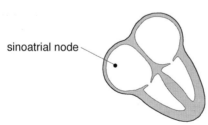

sinoatrial node

Fig. 3.1 The rhythm strip

Key points:
- rhythm strips are prolonged recordings from a single lead, often lead II
- this rhythm strip shows sinus rhythm

Even with a rhythm strip, however, the diagnosis of abnormal cardiac rhythms is not always easy, and some of the more complex arrhythmias can tax the skills of even the most experienced cardiologist. It is appropriate, therefore, to begin this chapter with the following warning.

> ⚡ **SEEK HELP**
>
> If in doubt about a patient's cardiac rhythm, do not hesitate to seek the advice of a cardiologist.

This advice is particularly important if the patient is haemodynamically compromised by the arrhythmia, or if you are contemplating treatment of any kind.

There are many ways in which one can approach the identification of arrhythmias, and this is reflected in the numerous ways in which they can be categorized:

- regular versus irregular
- bradycardias versus tachycardias
- narrow complex versus broad complex
- supraventricular versus ventricular.

The common cardiac rhythms are listed in Table 3.1. The first half of this chapter contains a brief description of each rhythm in turn, together with example ECGs. In the second half, 'Identifying the cardiac rhythm', we guide you towards the correct diagnosis of the cardiac rhythm.

● Common cardiac rhythms

Sinus rhythm

Sinus rhythm is the normal cardiac rhythm, in which the sinoatrial (SA) node acts as the natural pacemaker, discharging 60–100 times/min (Fig. 3.2).

Table 3.1 Cardiac rhythms

- SA nodal rhythms
  - sinus rhythm
  - sinus bradycardia
  - sinus tachycardia
  - sinus arrhythmia
  - sick sinus syndrome
- Atrial rhythms
  - atrial tachycardia
  - atrial flutter
  - atrial fibrillation
- AV junctional rhythms
- AV re-entry tachycardias
- Ventricular rhythms
  - ventricular tachycardia
  - accelerated idioventricular rhythm
  - torsades de pointes
  - ventricular fibrillation
- Conduction disturbances
- Escape rhythms
- Ectopic beats

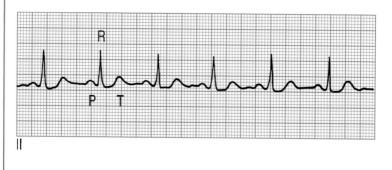

Fig. 3.2 Sinus rhythm

sinoatrial node

Key points:
- heart rate is 80 beats/min
- P waves are upright (lead II)
- QRS complex after every P wave

The characteristic features of sinus rhythm are:

- the heart rate is 60–100 beats/min
- the P wave is upright in lead II and inverted in lead aVR
- every P wave is followed by a QRS complex.

If the patient is in sinus rhythm, move on to determine the cardiac axis (Chapter 4). If not, continue reading this chapter to diagnose the rhythm.

Sinus bradycardia

Sinus bradycardia is sinus rhythm with a heart rate of less than 60 beats/min (Fig. 3.3).

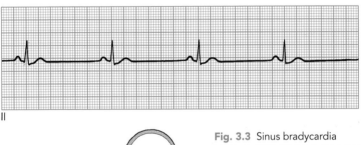

II

Fig. 3.3 Sinus bradycardia

Key points:
- heart rate is 43 beats/min
- P waves are upright (lead II)
- QRS complex after every P wave

sinoatrial node

The characteristic features of sinus bradycardia are:

- the heart rate is *less than* 60 beats/min
- the P wave is upright in lead II and inverted in lead aVR
- every P wave is followed by a QRS complex.

It is unusual for sinus bradycardia to be slower than 40 beats/min – any slower and you should consider an alternative cause, such as heart block (p. 119). Sinus bradycardia can be a normal finding, e.g. in athletes or during sleep. However, always consider the following possible causes:

- drugs (e.g. digoxin, beta blockers – including eye drops)
- ischaemic heart disease and myocardial infarction
- hypothyroidism
- hypothermia
- electrolyte abnormalities
- obstructive jaundice
- uraemia
- raised intracranial pressure
- sick sinus syndrome.

If the sinus bradycardia is severe, escape beats and escape rhythms may occur.

The management of bradycardia (of any cause) is discussed in Chapter 2.

Sinus tachycardia

Sinus tachycardia is sinus rhythm with a heart rate of greater than 100 beats/min (Fig. 3.4).

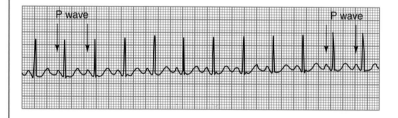

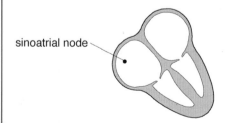

sinoatrial node

Fig. 3.4 Sinus tachycardia

Key points:
- heart rate is 138 beats/min
- P waves are upright (lead II)
- QRS complex after every P wave

The characteristic features of sinus tachycardia are:

- the heart rate is *greater than* 100 beats/min
- the P wave is upright in lead II and inverted in lead aVR
- every P wave is followed by a QRS complex.

It is rare for sinus tachycardia to exceed 180 beats/min, except in fit athletes. At this heart rate, it may be difficult to differentiate the P waves from the T waves, so the rhythm can be mistaken for an atrioventricular (AV) nodal re-entry tachycardia.

Physiological causes of sinus tachycardia include anything that stimulates the sympathetic nervous system – anxiety, pain, fear, fever or exercise. Always consider the following causes as well:

- drugs, e.g. adrenaline, atropine, salbutamol (do not forget inhalers and nebulizers), caffeine and alcohol
- ischaemic heart disease and acute myocardial infarction
- heart failure
- pulmonary embolism
- fluid loss
- anaemia
- hyperthyroidism.

The management of sinus tachycardia is that of the cause. When a patient has an **appropriate** tachycardia (compensating for low blood pressure, such as in fluid loss or anaemia), slowing it with beta blockers can lead to disastrous decompensation. It is the underlying problem that needs addressing. However, if the sinus tachycardia is **inappropriate**, as in anxiety or hyperthyroidism, treatment with beta blockers may be helpful.

> **! WARNING**
>
> In sinus tachycardia, never use a beta blocker to slow the heart rate until you have established the cause.

Persistent 'sinus tachycardia' should lead to suspicion that the diagnosis may be incorrect – both atrial flutter and atrial tachycardia can, on casual inspection, be mistaken for sinus tachycardia. However, persistent 'inappropriate' sinus tachycardia is recognized as a clinical entity, referring to a resting heart rate above 100 beats/min (in sinus rhythm), but the condition is poorly understood. It may result from enhanced automaticity within the SA node or from autonomic dysfunction. Inappropriate sinus tachycardia can be treated with rate-controlling drugs (such as beta blockers) or, in severe symptomatic cases, electrophysiological modification/ablation of the SA node.

Sinus arrhythmia

Sinus arrhythmia is the variation in heart rate that is seen during inspiration and expiration (Fig. 3.5).

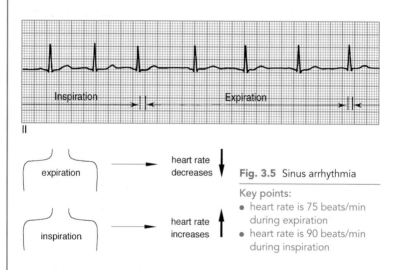

Fig. 3.5 Sinus arrhythmia

Key points:
- heart rate is 75 beats/min during expiration
- heart rate is 90 beats/min during inspiration

The characteristic features of sinus arrhythmia are:

- every P wave is followed by a QRS complex
- the heart rate varies with respiration.

The heart rate normally increases during inspiration, as a reflex response to the increased volume of blood returning to the heart. Sinus arrhythmia is uncommon after the age of

40 years. The condition is harmless and no tests or treatment are necessary.

Sick sinus syndrome

As the name suggests, sick sinus syndrome is a collection of impulse generation and conduction problems related to dysfunction of the sinus node. Any, or all, of the following problems may be seen in a patient with the syndrome:

- sinus bradycardia
- sinus arrest
- SA block.

Sinus bradycardia has already been described (p. 31). The sinus node is normally a very reliable pacemaker. However, in **sinus arrest**, it sometimes fails to discharge on time – looking at a rhythm strip, a P wave will suddenly fail to appear in the expected place, and there is a gap, of variable length, until the sinus node fires and a P wave appears, or a junctional escape beat is generated by a 'safety net' subsidiary pacemaker in the AV junction (Fig. 3.6).

P wave fails to appear

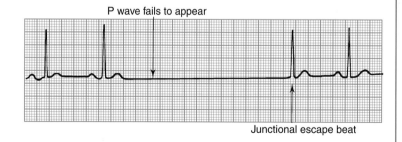

Junctional escape beat

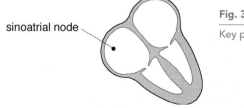

sinoatrial node

Fig. 3.6 Sinus arrest

Key points:
- P wave fails to appear
- next P wave does not appear where expected

In an **SA block**, the sinus node depolarizes as normal, but the impulse fails to reach the atria. A P wave fails to appear in the expected place, but the next one usually appears exactly where it is expected (Fig. 3.7).

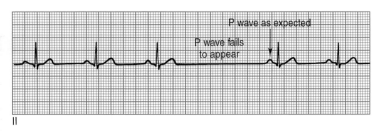

P wave as expected

P wave fails to appear

II

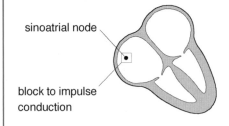

sinoatrial node

block to impulse conduction

Fig. 3.7 Sinoatrial block

Key points:
- P wave fails to appear
- next P wave appears where expected

If the sinus bradycardia is severe, or if sinus arrest or SA block is prolonged, escape beats and escape rhythms (p. 59) may occur. Sick sinus syndrome may also coexist with:

- certain paroxysmal tachycardias
  - atrial tachycardia (p. 37)
  - atrial flutter (p. 39)
  - atrial fibrillation (AF) (p. 42)
- AV nodal conduction disorders (p. 119).

The association of sick sinus syndrome with paroxysmal tachy-cardias is called **tachycardia–bradycardia (or 'tachy-brady') syndrome**. The tachycardias often emerge as an escape rhythm in response to an episode of bradycardia. Evidence for abnormal AV nodal conduction often becomes apparent when a patient with tachy-brady syndrome develops AF with a slow ventricular response – the AV node fails to conduct the atrial impulses at the usual high rate.

Sick sinus syndrome, and the associated tachy-brady syndrome, may cause symptoms of dizziness, fainting and palpitations. The commonest cause of sick sinus syndrome is degeneration and fibrosis of the sinus node and conducting system. Other causes to consider are:

- ischaemic heart disease
- drugs (e.g. beta blockers, digoxin, quinidine)
- cardiomyopathy
- amyloidosis
- myocarditis.

The diagnosis usually requires a 24-h ambulatory ECG recording, also known as **Holter monitoring** (see Chapter 15).

Asymptomatic patients do not require treatment. Patients with symptoms need consideration for a permanent pacemaker (Chapter 14). This is particularly important if they also have paroxysmal tachycardias that require anti-arrhythmic drugs (which can worsen the episodes of bradycardia). Paroxysmal tachycardias that arise as escape rhythms in response to episodes of bradycardia may also improve as a consequence of pacing. Referral to a cardiologist is therefore recommended.

Atrial tachycardia

Atrial tachycardia differs from sinus tachycardia in that the impulses are generated by an ectopic focus somewhere within the atrial myocardium rather than the sinus node (Fig. 3.8). More than one focus may be present in any one patient (multifocal atrial tachycardia), giving rise to several P wave morphologies.

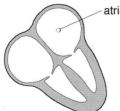

atrial ectopic focus

Fig. 3.8 Abnormal atrial focus

Key point:
- the abnormal focus means the spread of depolarization through the atria follows an abnormal route

Atrial tachycardia results in a rhythm strip with the following characteristic features (Fig. 3.9):

- heart rate greater than 100 beats/min
- abnormally shaped P waves.

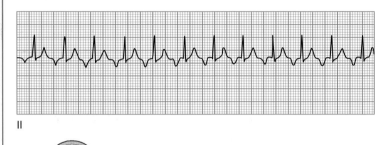

II

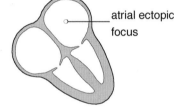

atrial ectopic focus

Fig. 3.9 Atrial tachycardia

Key points:
- heart rate is 125 beats/min
- abnormally shaped P waves

The atrial (P wave) rate is usually 120–250/min; above atrial rates of 200/min, the AV node struggles to keep up with impulse conduction and AV block may occur. The combination of atrial tachycardia with AV block is particularly common in digoxin toxicity. If the patient is not taking digoxin, consider:

- ischaemic heart disease
- chronic obstructive pulmonary disease
- rheumatic heart disease
- cardiomyopathy
- sick sinus syndrome (p. 35).

For details on how to manage digoxin toxicity, see the section on digoxin in Chapter 9 (p. 180). If digoxin is not the cause, it can be used to control the ventricular response, as can a beta blocker or verapamil.

> **! WARNING**
>
> Never give verapamil to a patient who is taking a beta blocker (or vice versa). A severe bradycardia can result.

Atrial flutter

Atrial flutter usually results from a re-entry circuit within the right atrium. It takes about 0.2 s for the impulse to complete a circuit of the right atrium (in most cases moving in an anticlockwise direction), giving rise to a wave of depolarization across both atria and a flutter wave on the ECG. There are thus about 5 flutter waves every second, and around 300 every minute (Fig. 3.10).

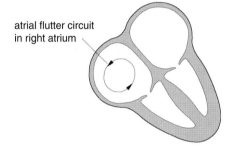

atrial flutter circuit
in right atrium

Fig. 3.10 Atrial flutter circuit

Key points: • a circuit of activity circles the right atrium

In atrial flutter the atrial rate is usually 250–350/min and often almost exactly 300/min. The AV node cannot keep up with such a high atrial rate and AV block occurs. This is most commonly 2:1 block, where only alternate atrial impulses get through the AV node to initiate a QRS complex, although 3:1, 4:1 or variable degrees of block are also seen (Fig. 3.11).

Thus, the ventricular rate is less than the atrial rate, and is often 150, 100 or 75/min. You should always suspect atrial flutter with 2:1 block when a patient has a regular tachycardia with a ventricular rate of about 150/min.

The rapid atrial rate gives a characteristic 'sawtooth' appearance to the baseline of the ECG, made up of flutter or 'F' waves. This can be made more apparent by carotid sinus massage or by giving adenosine. This will not terminate the atrial flutter, but will

39

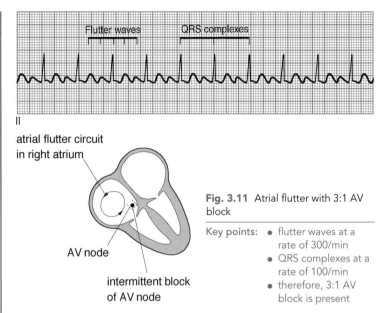

Flutter waves   QRS complexes

II

atrial flutter circuit
in right atrium

AV node

intermittent block
of AV node

Fig. 3.11 Atrial flutter with 3:1 AV block

Key points:
- flutter waves at a rate of 300/min
- QRS complexes at a rate of 100/min
- therefore, 3:1 AV block is present

increase the degree of AV block, making the baseline easier to see by reducing the number of QRS complexes (Fig. 3.12). Carotid sinus massage should be performed with the patient supine and with the neck slightly extended. Do not perform carotid sinus massage if carotid bruits are present, or if there is a history of cerebral thromboembolism. Massage the carotid artery on one side of the neck, medial to the sternomastoid muscle, for 5 s. The technique can be repeated, if necessary, on the opposite side after waiting for 1 min. The ECG must be monitored continuously throughout the procedure.

Thus, the characteristic features of atrial flutter are:

- atrial rate around 300/min
- 'sawtooth' baseline
- AV block (commonly 2:1, but can be 3:1, 4:1 or variable).

The causes of atrial flutter are the same as those of AF (see Table 3.2). Although beta blockers, verapamil or digoxin can be used simply to control the ventricular response, it is preferable

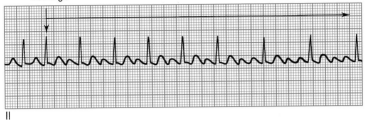

Carotid sinus massage

II

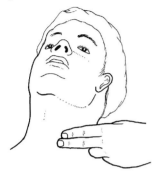

Fig. 3.12 The effect of carotid sinus massage

Key points:
- carotid sinus massage increases the degree of AV block
- the QRS rate falls from 100/min to 75/min
- the flutter waves are more easily seen when there are fewer QRS complexes

to aim to restore sinus rhythm. Drugs that can restore (and maintain) sinus rhythm include:

- sotalol
- flecainide
- amiodarone.

Table 3.2 Causes of atrial fibrillation

- Hypertension
- Ischaemic heart disease
- Hyperthyroidism
- Sick sinus syndrome
- Alcohol
- Rheumatic mitral valve disease
- Cardiomyopathy
- Atrial septal defect
- Pericarditis
- Myocarditis
- Pulmonary embolism
- Pneumonia
- Cardiac surgery
- Idiopathic ('lone') atrial fibrillation

Atrial flutter can also be converted to sinus rhythm with direct current (DC) cardioversion (p. 45) and overdrive atrial pacing (Chapter 14). Atrial flutter ablation can be used to prevent recurrence of the arrhythmia. This is an electrophysiological technique in which the re-entry circuit is identified in the right atrium and a section of it is permanently ablated using diathermy to 'break' the circuit underlying the re-entry loop. Atrial flutter carries a risk of thromboembolism, and patients with atrial flutter are usually considered for antiplatelet drugs or anticoagulation according to the guidelines similar to those used in AF (see below).

Atrial fibrillation

Atrial fibrillation is much commoner than atrial flutter, affecting 5–10 per cent of elderly people. It can be classified as:

- **paroxysmal AF** – spontaneously terminating episodes of AF on a background of sinus rhythm
- **persistent AF** – continuous AF with no intervening sinus rhythm
- **permanent AF** – continuous AF where there is no expectation of restoring sinus rhythm (e.g. by DC cardioversion).

The basis of AF is rapid, chaotic depolarization occurring throughout the atria as a consequence of multiple 'wavelets' of activation. No P waves are seen and the ECG baseline consists of low-amplitude oscillations (fibrillation or 'f' waves). Although around 350–600 impulses reach the AV node every minute, only 120–180 of these will reach the ventricles to produce QRS complexes. Transmission of the atrial impulses through the AV node is erratic, making the ventricular (QRS complex) rhythm 'irregularly irregular' (Fig. 3.13).

Thus, the characteristic features of AF are:

- absence of P waves
- irregularly irregular ventricular rhythm.

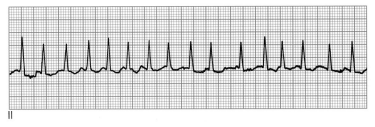

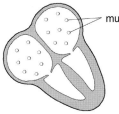

multiple atrial foci

Fig. 3.13 Atrial fibrillation

Key points:
- irregularly irregular rhythm
- no P waves visible
- QRS rate is 170/min

The erratic atrial depolarization leads to a failure of effective atrial contraction. Loss of the 'atrial kick' reduces ventricular filling and can lead to a fall of 10–15 per cent in cardiac output.

Patients with AF usually present with palpitations and/or symptoms of an underlying cause (Table 3.2). Systemic embolism is an important risk in AF and may also be a presenting feature. Examination of the patient will reveal an irregularly irregular pulse.

Once AF has been diagnosed, a cause should be sought with a thorough patient history and examination. Thyroid function tests are essential, as AF may be the only sign of a thyroid disorder. Echocardiography may also be helpful. Treatment of an underlying cause can resolve the arrhythmia.

In treating permanent AF, aim to:

- control the ventricular rate
- reduce the risk of thromboembolism
- restore sinus rhythm where appropriate.

Rate control is achieved with AV nodal blocking drugs, such as beta blockers, verapamil or digoxin.

> **! WARNING**
>
> Never give verapamil to a patient who is taking a beta blocker (or vice versa). A severe bradycardia can result.

In the UK, the National Institute for Health and Clinical Excellence (NICE) issued helpful guidelines on AF management in 2006, which included an algorithm for decision making about aspirin versus warfarin. The risk of stroke in AF is reduced by about 60 per cent with anticoagulation treatment using warfarin and by about 25 per cent with aspirin. Risk factors that place patients with AF at high risk of stroke include:

- previous stroke or thromboembolic event
- age ⩾75 years with coexistent hypertension, diabetes or vascular disease
- clinical evidence of valve disease or heart failure (or impaired left ventricular function on echo).

These patients should be considered for anticoagulation with warfarin, in the absence of any contraindications. Patients aged ⩾65 years with none of these high-risk factors, or those aged <75 years with hypertension, diabetes or vascular disease, are at moderate risk of stroke and can be considered for either warfarin or aspirin. Patients aged <65 years with no high or moderate risk factors are at low risk of stroke and can be treated with aspirin 75–300 mg daily (if no contraindications).

According to the NICE guidance, attempts to restore sinus rhythm through either DC cardioversion or pharmacological cardioversion are appropriate for patients who:

- have symptoms with their AF
- are younger
- are presenting for the first time with lone AF
- have AF secondary to a corrected precipitant
- have heart failure.

● Direct current cardioversion for atrial fibrillation

Although DC cardioversion for AF is often initially successful in restoring sinus rhythm, the arrhythmia frequently recurs. Long-term success is more likely if patients have been in AF for only a short time and if the atria are not significantly enlarged.

Four weeks of full anticoagulation prior to elective DC cardioversion reduces thromboembolic risk. Oral digoxin need not be routinely stopped prior to the procedure, although there is a risk of precipitating a ventricular arrhythmia if digoxin toxicity is present.

Patients must be 'nil by mouth' on the day of the procedure as they will require general anaesthesia. Check their electrolyte levels and international normalized ratio (INR). The patient should be fully anticoagulated and the plasma potassium level should be ≥ 4 mmol/L. If there is a possibility of digoxin toxicity (suggested by symptoms, ECG findings, high dosage or renal impairment), check the patient's digoxin level.

The technique of giving a DC shock is described in Chapter 17. Set the defibrillator to synchronized mode and start at an energy level of 100 J, increasing to 200 J and 360 J as appropriate. In atrial flutter, start at a lower energy level of 50 J. Biphasic defibrillators also require lower energy levels.

If cardioversion is successful, continue anticoagulation and review the patient after 4 weeks in clinic. If they are still in sinus rhythm, anticoagulation can be discontinued.

Conversely, control of ventricular rate (rather than cardioversion back to sinus rhythm) is considered more appropriate in patients with:

● age >65 years
● coronary artery disease

- contraindications to antiarrhythmic drugs or anticoagulation
- a large left atrium (>5.5 cm)
- mitral stenosis
- >12 months duration of AF
- multiple failed attempts at cardioversion or relapses
- an ongoing reversible cause for AF (such as thyrotoxicosis).

A permanent restoration of sinus rhythm can be difficult to achieve, particularly in patients who have been in AF for a long time. Certain drugs (sotalol, flecainide, amiodarone) can restore sinus rhythm, as can DC cardioversion (see box above). Maintenance of sinus rhythm can be achieved with any of these drugs, but there is only around a 50:50 chance of sustaining sinus rhythm beyond 1 year. Amiodarone is probably more effective, but can have troublesome side effects, including thyroid and liver dysfunction, pulmonary toxicity, reversible corneal microdeposits, skin discoloration and photosensitivity.

In paroxysmal AF, the aim should be to reduce the risk of embolization (as above) and to reduce the likelihood of recurrent paroxysms. Sotalol, flecainide or amiodarone may be useful. Digoxin should be avoided as it does not help in paroxysmal AF and may even make it worse.

Patients whose AF is resistant to treatment should be referred to a cardiologist.

AV re-entry tachycardias

AV re-entry tachycardias can arise when there is a second connection between the atria and ventricles, in addition to the normal route of conduction via the AV node. The presence of two different routes creates the possibility that impulses can travel down one (anterograde conduction) and then back up the other (retrograde conduction). In doing so, an impulse can enter into a repeated cycle of activity, circling round the two pathways so that it repeatedly re-enters and activates the atria and ventricles in rapid succession (Fig. 3.14).

● Resistant atrial fibrillation

The non-pharmacological treatment of resistant AF includes:

- pulmonary vein isolation (to prevent ectopic beats arising within the pulmonary veins from reaching the left atrium and acting as a trigger for atrial fibrillation)
- AV nodal ablation (to prevent conduction from the atria to the ventricles) with insertion of a permanent ventricular pacemaker
- experimental surgical techniques to remodel the atrial myocardium to redirect the flow of atrial impulses.

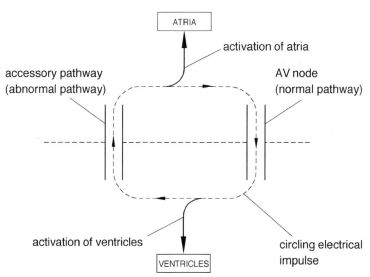

Fig. 3.14 Conduction circling around an AV re-entry circuit

The extra connection between the atria and ventricles can be either an **accessory pathway**, anatomically separate from the AV node, or a **dual AV nodal pathway**, in which both pathways lie within the AV node but are electrically distinct (Fig. 3.15).

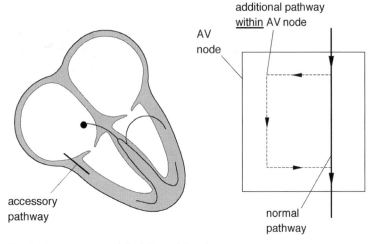

additional pathway
within AV node

AV
node

accessory
pathway

normal
pathway

Fig. 3.15 Accessory and dual AV nodal pathways

Accessory pathways are found in the Wolff–Parkinson–White (WPW) syndrome (described in Chapter 6) and patients are susceptible to episodes of **AV re-entry tachycardia**, with anterograde conduction via the AV node and retrograde conduction via the accessory pathway. During the tachycardia the delta wave is lost (Fig. 3.16). A re-entrant tachycardia taking the opposite route (down the accessory pathway and up the AV node) is rare, but when it does occur, only delta waves are seen (as the whole of the ventricular muscle is activated via the accessory pathway).

Patients with a dual AV nodal pathway are at risk of **AV nodal re-entry tachycardia**. One of the AV nodal pathways conducts impulses quickly (the 'fast' pathway) but has a long refractory period. The other AV nodal pathway conducts impulses more slowly (the 'slow' pathway) but has a shorter refractory period. Normally, an impulse arriving at the AV node will split and travel down both pathways at the same time, but the impulse travelling via the fast pathway arrives, as one would expect, at the bundle of His first and goes on to

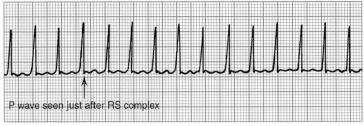

P wave seen just after RS complex

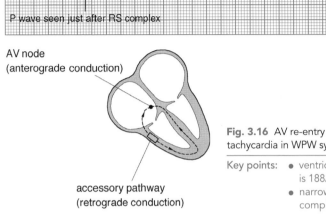

AV node
(anterograde conduction)

accessory pathway
(retrograde conduction)

Fig. 3.16 AV re-entry
tachycardia in WPW syndrome

Key points:
- ventricular rate is 188/min
- narrow RS complexes

depolarize the ventricles. By the time that the impulse travelling down the slow pathway arrives at the bundle of His, the bundle is refractory and so this impulse goes no further.

However, if a supraventricular ectopic beat happens to occur during the refractory period of the fast pathway, this ectopic will travel down the slow pathway and, by the time it reaches the end of the slow pathway, the fast pathway may have repolarized. If so, this impulse will then travel back *up* along the fast pathway, and then back down the slow pathway, *ad infinitum*. This re-entry circuit is what gives rise to an AV nodal re-entry tachycardia (Fig. 3.17).

Both AV re-entry tachycardia and AV nodal re-entry tachycardia have the following characteristics:

- the heart rate is 130–250 beats/min
- there is one P wave per QRS complex (although P waves are not always clearly seen)

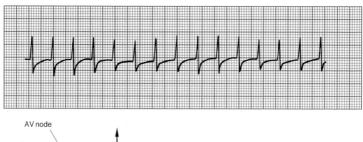

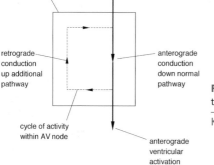

AV node

retrograde
conduction
up additional
pathway

anterograde
conduction
down normal
pathway

cycle of activity
within AV node

anterograde
ventricular
activation

Fig. 3.17 AV nodal re-entry tachycardia

Key points:
- ventricular rate is 180/min
- narrow RS complexes

- there are regular QRS complexes
- QRS complexes are narrow (in the absence of aberrant conduction).

The QRS complexes will be broad if there is pre-existing or rate-dependent bundle branch block. The rhythm can then be mistaken for ventricular tachycardia (VT) (p. 53). An earlier ECG, if available, may be helpful in determining whether a bundle branch block existed before the tachycardia.

In AV re-entry tachycardia, inverted P waves (p. 105) are often seen halfway between QRS complexes. In AV nodal re-entry tachycardia, the inverted P waves are often harder or even impossible to discern as they follow the QRS complexes closely or are buried within them.

Although the position of the P waves may help distinguish between AV re-entry tachycardia and AV nodal re-entry tachycardia, an ECG in sinus rhythm is more helpful as it may reveal a short PR interval or delta wave, suggesting WPW syndrome (p. 114). The definite diagnosis can be difficult, however, and sometimes requires electrophysiological studies.

Symptoms of AV re-entry tachycardias vary greatly between patients. Palpitations is the commonest complaint but can vary greatly in duration and severity. Palpitations start suddenly and may be accompanied by chest pain, dizziness or syncope.

AV re-entry tachycardias can be terminated by blocking the AV node, thereby breaking the cycle of electrical activity. The **Valsalva manoeuvre** increases vagal inhibition of AV nodal conduction, thus slowing the AV nodal conduction and often terminating the tachycardia. Alternatively, you can perform **carotid sinus massage** (while monitoring the ECG) with the same aim, as long as the patient does not have carotid bruits. The technique of carotid sinus massage is described on page 40.

● Valsalva manoeuvre

The Valsalva manoeuvre describes the action of forced expiration against a closed glottis. To perform it, patients should be asked to breathe in and then to strain for a few seconds with their breath held. Alternatively, they can be given a 20 mL plastic syringe and asked to 'blow' into the hole to try to push out the plunger from the opposite end. This is impossible to achieve, but in trying to do so the patient effectively performs a Valsalva manoeuvre.

Drug treatments include intravenous adenosine (do not use if the patient has asthma or obstructive airways disease) or intravenous verapamil (not to be used if the patient has recently taken a beta blocker). If the patient is haemodynamically compromised, consider urgent **DC cardioversion** (p. 45) or **overdrive atrial pacing** (Chapter 14).

 WARNING

Never give verapamil to a patient who is taking a beta blocker (or vice versa). A severe bradycardia can result.

In the longer term, the arrhythmia does not require prophylactic treatment if episodes are brief and cause few symptoms. Patients can be taught to use the Valsalva manoeuvre. If drug treatment is required, referral to a cardiologist is recommended. Sotalol is often effective as a first-line agent, but radiofrequency ablation via a cardiac catheter can be curative.

● Atrial fibrillation in Wolff–Parkinson–White syndrome

AV re-entry tachycardia is not the only arrhythmia seen in WPW syndrome. Atrial fibrillation can be precipitated by the re-entry tachycardia. If the patient goes into AF, conduction to the ventricles can occur via either the accessory pathway (which is commonest) or the AV node, or both. Conduction via the accessory pathway can cause a rapid and potentially lethal ventricular rate in response. Drugs that block the AV node (e.g. digoxin, verapamil or adenosine) are therefore hazardous in these patients, as they will increase conduction down the accessory pathway. Direct current cardioversion is the treatment of choice if the patient is haemodynamically compromised. Recurrent episodes can be treated with drugs that slow conduction in the accessory pathway, such as amiodarone. Patients who have had AF in WPV syndrome should be considered for accessory pathway ablation.

Ventricular tachycardia

Ventricular tachycardia is a **broad-complex tachycardia**, defined as three or more successive ventricular beats at a heart rate above 120 beats/min. It arises either from a re-entry circuit or from increased automaticity of a specific ventricular focus. Episodes can be self-terminating or sustained (defined as lasting longer than 30 s), and can also degenerate into VF (Fig. 3.18).

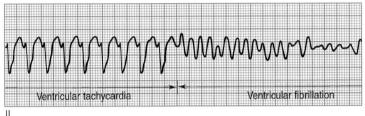

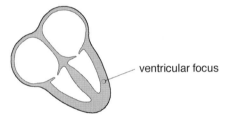

ventricular focus

Fig. 3.18 Ventricular tachycardia (VT) and ventricular fibrillation (VF)

Key points:
- broad-complex tachycardia at a rate of 190/min (VT)
- degenerates into chaotic rhythm (VF)

Characteristic features of VT are:

- ventricular rate above 120/min
- broad QRS complexes.

Sustained VT usually occurs at a heart rate of 150–250/min, but the diagnosis can be difficult. Ventricular tachycardia can be well tolerated and may not cause haemodynamic disturbance. Do *not* assume, therefore, that just because the patient appears well, they do not have VT. See the section 'Identifying a cardiac rhythm' below for help with distinguishing VT from arrhythmias with similar ECG appearances.

The symptoms of VT can vary from mild palpitations to dizziness, syncope and cardiac arrest. Always look for an underlying treatable cause (Table 3.3).

Table 3.3 Causes of ventricular tachycardia

- Acute myocardial infarction
- Ischaemic heart disease
- Hypertrophic cardiomyopathy
- Dilated cardiomyopathy
- Arrhythmogenic right ventricular cardiomyopathy
- Long QT syndrome
- Myocarditis
- Congenital heart disease (repaired or unrepaired)
- Electrolyte disturbance
- Pro-arrhythmic drugs
- Mitral valve prolapse
- Idiopathic (e.g. right ventricular outflow tract tachycardia)

An episode of VT can be terminated using:

- drugs
- DC cardioversion
- pacing.

Choose the treatment according to the clinical state of the patient. When haemodynamic impairment is present, VT becomes a medical emergency and warrants urgent DC cardioversion (Chapter 17).

 ACT QUICKLY

Ventricular tachycardia causing haemodynamic compromise is an emergency. Immediate diagnosis and treatment are required.

Stable patients can be cardioverted medically. Amiodarone is often the first-line agent, but alternatives include lidocaine (lignocaine), flecainide and sotalol. Overdrive right ventricular pacing (Chapter 14) is also effective but may precipitate VF.

Long-term prophylaxis should be discussed with a cardiologist. Usually it is not necessary for VT occurring within the first 48 h following an acute myocardial infarction. Effective drug treatments include sotalol (particularly when VT is exercise related) and amiodarone. Ventricular tachycardia related to bradycardia should be treated by pacing. Ablation or surgery can be used to remove a ventricular focus or re-entry circuit identified by electrophysiological testing. Finally, implantable cardioverter defibrillator devices (ICDs) can be implanted to deliver overdrive pacing and/or low-energy DC shocks for recurrent episodes of VT and VF (see Chapter 14).

VT can also be idiopathic in the context of an apparently structurally normal heart. The most common type is right ventricular outflow tract (RVOT) tachycardia, which accounts for around 10 per cent of all forms of VT. It is often seen in association with ventricular ectopic beats, which have a characteristic appearance of left bundle branch block and an inferior axis indicative of their RVOT origin. Exercise and emotional stress can trigger RVOT ectopics and also RVOT tachycardia, but nonetheless the prognosis for these patients is generally good. It is important, however, not to mistake the relatively benign RVOT form of VT with VT caused by arrhythmogenic right ventricular cardiomyopathy (ARVC), which has a more sinister prognosis. In ARVC the heart is not structurally normal, and the abnormal right ventricular morphology can be identified by echocardiography or cardiac magnetic resonance imaging. Ventricular tachycardia in the context of ARVC is treated with an ICD, whereas symptomatic RVOT tachycardia is usually treated with ablation.

The polymorphic variant of VT (torsades de pointes) is discussed below.

SEEK HELP

The management options for VT should be discussed with a cardiologist.

Accelerated idioventricular rhythm

Accelerated idioventricular rhythm is a slow form of VT, with a heart rate of less than 120 beats/min (Fig. 3.19).

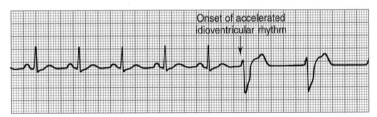

Onset of accelerated idioventricular rhythm

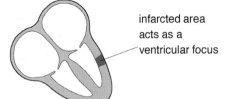

infarcted area acts as a ventricular focus

Fig. 3.19 Accelerated idioventricular rhythm

Key points:
- broad QRS complexes
- heart rate is 60 beats/min

It is usually seen in the setting of an acute myocardial infarction and is benign. No treatment is necessary.

Torsades de pointes (polymorphic VT)

Torsades de pointes is a variant of VT that is polymorphic and is associated with a long QT interval (p. 207). Its name derives from the characteristic undulating pattern on the ECG, with a variation in the direction of the QRS axis (Fig. 3.20).

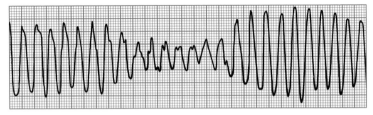

II

Fig. 3.20 Torsades de pointes

Key points:
- broad-complex tachycardia (rate is 270/min)
- variation in QRS axis

Torsades de pointes can occur with hereditary long QT syndromes (see Chapter 11), certain anti-arrhythmic drug treatments (and drug interactions), and electrolyte abnormalities (hypokalaemia and hypomagnesaemia). As it carries a risk of precipitating VF, urgent assessment is warranted, with referral to a cardiologist if necessary. Any causative drugs need to be identified and withdrawn, and electrolyte abnormalities corrected.

In an emergency, standard adult life support protocols (see Chapter 17) should be followed. Torsades de pointes can be treated by giving magnesium (which is often effective even if the magnesium level is normal) and correcting any other electrolyte abnormalities. Any drugs that can prolong the QT interval should be withdrawn. Temporary pacing, which increases the heart rate and thereby shortens the QT interval, can be helpful. In the congenital long QT syndromes, left cervical sympathectomy can sometimes be indicated to interrupt the sympathetic supply to the heart. An ICD may be required if the patient is judged to be at high risk of sudden cardiac death.

> **SEEK HELP**
>
> Torsades de pointes can cause VF. Urgent referral to a cardiologist is recommended.

Ventricular fibrillation

Untreated VF is a rapidly fatal arrhythmia. It therefore requires immediate diagnosis and treatment. See Chapter 17 for the emergency management algorithm for this arrhythmia (p. 256).

Ventricular fibrillation is most commonly seen in the setting of an acute myocardial infarction. Always check for electrolyte or acid–base abnormalities following an episode of VF. A single episode of **primary VF** (occurring within 48 h of an infarction), once corrected by DC shock, does not require prophylactic treatment.

Recurrent episodes of VF, or **secondary VF** (after 48 h), merit prophylaxis with amiodarone, beta blockers or lidocaine. Long-term prophylaxis is the same as for VT.

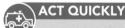

ACT QUICKLY

Ventricular fibrillation is a medical emergency.
Immediate diagnosis and treatment are essential.

Conduction disturbances

The normal conduction of impulses from the SA node to the ventricles is described in Chapter 1. A block can occur at different points along this route (Fig. 3.21).

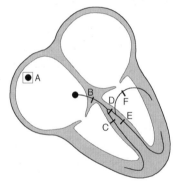

A: Sinoatrial block
B: Atrioventricular block
C: Right bundle branch block
D: Left bundle branch block
E: Left posterior fascicular hemiblock
F: Left anterior fascicular hemiblock

Fig. 3.21 Regions where conduction blocks can occur

In **sinoatrial block**, the SA node depolarizes as normal, but the impulse fails to reach the atria. A P wave fails to appear in the expected place, but the next one usually appears exactly on time. An example is shown in Figure 3.7.

Atrioventricular block (Chapter 6) has three degrees of severity. First-degree AV block simply lengthens the PR interval by delaying conduction through the AV node. In second-degree AV block, some atrial impulses fail to be conducted to the ventricles. In third-degree AV block, there is no conduction between atria and ventricles.

Further down the conducting system, **bundle branch block** can affect either the left or right bundle branch. Sometimes only one of the two fascicles of the left bundle branch is affected. Any permutation of these is possible, and block of both bundle branches together is equivalent to third-degree AV block, as no impulses will reach the ventricular myocardium. Bundle branch block is discussed on page 147, and fascicular block on pages 92 and 98.

Conduction disturbances are not always a consistent feature of the ECG. They can be rate dependent, only appearing at high heart rates when compromised regions of the conducting system fail to keep pace with the conduction of impulses. The development of bundle branch block during a supraventricular tachycardia (SVT), for example, can give it the appearance of VT (p. 74).

Conduction disturbances are important to recognize, not only because of their effects on the appearance of the ECG but also because escape rhythms can appear when there is complete block of normal conduction.

Escape rhythms

Escape rhythms are a form of 'safety net' for the heart. Without escape rhythms, complete failure of impulse generation or conduction at any time would lead to ventricular asystole and death. Instead, the heart has a number of subsidiary pacemakers that can take over if normal impulse generation or conduction fails.

The subsidiary pacemakers are located in the AV junction and the ventricular myocardium. If the AV junction fails to receive impulses, as a result of SA arrest or block, or even during severe sinus bradycardia, it will take over as the cardiac pacemaker. The QRS complex(es) generated will have the same morphology as normal, but at a slower rate of around 40–60 beats/min (Fig. 3.22).

The AV junctional pacemaker will continue until it again starts to be inhibited by impulses from the SA node. If the AV junctional

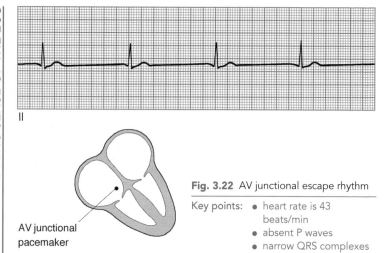

Fig. 3.22 AV junctional escape rhythm

AV junctional pacemaker

Key points:
- heart rate is 43 beats/min
- absent P waves
- narrow QRS complexes

pacemaker fails, or its impulses are blocked, a ventricular pacemaker will take over. Its rhythm is even slower, at 15–40 beats/min, and the QRS complexes will be broad (Fig. 3.23).

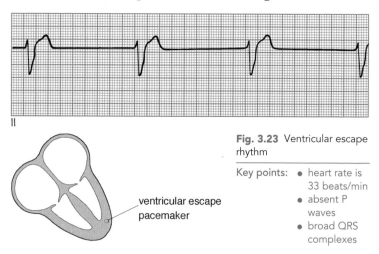

Fig. 3.23 Ventricular escape rhythm

ventricular escape pacemaker

Key points:
- heart rate is 33 beats/min
- absent P waves
- broad QRS complexes

Because escape rhythms exist as a safety net, they must *not* be suppressed. Instead, you must identify why the escape rhythm has arisen (i.e. why normal impulse generation has failed or been blocked) and correct that underlying problem. This will usually require a pacemaker and should be discussed with a cardiologist.

Ectopic beats

In contrast with the QRS complexes of escape rhythms, which appear *later* than expected, ectopic beats appear *earlier* than expected. They can arise from any region of the heart, but are usually classified into atrial, AV junctional and ventricular ectopics. Ectopic beats are also called **extrasystoles** and **premature beats**.

Atrial ectopics are identified by a P wave that appears earlier than expected and has an abnormal shape (Fig. 3.24). Although atrial ectopic beats will usually be conducted to the ventricles and give rise to a QRS complex, occasionally they may encounter a refractory AV node and fail to be conducted.

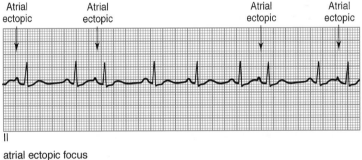

Atrial ectopic   Atrial ectopic   Atrial ectopic   Atrial ectopic

II

atrial ectopic focus

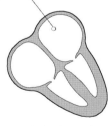

Fig. 3.24 Atrial ectopic beats

Key points: • P waves earlier than expected
           • P wave abnormally shaped

AV junctional ectopics will activate the ventricles, giving rise to a QRS complex earlier than expected (Fig. 3.25). They may also retrogradely activate the atria to cause an inverted P wave.

Whether the P wave occurs before, during or after the QRS complex simply depends on whether the electrical impulse reaches the atria or ventricles first.

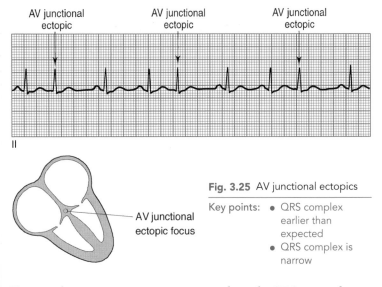

Fig. 3.25 AV junctional ectopics

Key points:
- QRS complex earlier than expected
- QRS complex is narrow

Ventricular ectopics give rise to broad QRS complexes. Occasionally, they will be followed by inverted P waves if the atria are activated by retrograde conduction. If retrograde conduction does not occur, there will usually be a full compensatory pause before the next normal beat because the SA node will not be 'reset' (Fig. 3.26).

Ventricular ectopics can occur at the same time as the T wave of the preceding beat. In the setting of an acute myocardial infarction, such 'R on T' ectopics can trigger ventricular arrhythmias.

Ventricular ectopics can be frequent. When one ectopic follows every normal beat, the term 'bigeminy' is used (Fig. 3.27). Ventricular ectopics can be harmless, particularly when the heart is structurally normal, but can also be associated with more hazardous arrhythmias, especially when heart disease is present. The assessment of the patient with ventricular ectopics should therefore include a search for any underlying

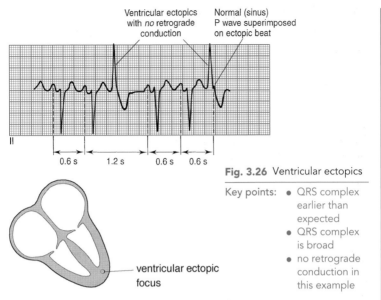

Ventricular ectopics with *no* retrograde conduction

Normal (sinus) P wave superimposed on ectopic beat

II

0.6 s   1.2 s   0.6 s   0.6 s

ventricular ectopic focus

Fig. 3.26 Ventricular ectopics

Key points:
- QRS complex earlier than expected
- QRS complex is broad
- no retrograde conduction in this example

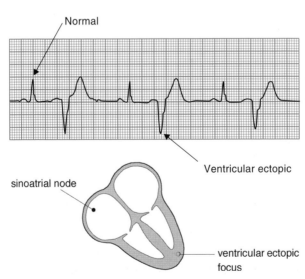

Normal

sinoatrial node

Ventricular ectopic

ventricular ectopic focus

Fig. 3.27 Bigeminy

Key point:
- each normal beat is followed by a ventricular ectopic

heart disease, which may include (in addition to a 12-lead ECG) echocardiography, exercise treadmill testing and ambulatory ECG monitoring.

Ventricular ectopics that arise from the RVOT are identified by their left bundle branch block morphology with an inferior axis on the ECG. Although this group of RVOT ectopics can be associated with non-sustained VT, they have traditionally been regarded as being associated with a generally good prognosis (although this assumption has been challenged, and many cases have been reported in which malignant ventricular arrhythmias have occurred). Right ventricular outflow tract ectopics should not be confused with the similar ventricular ectopics that are seen in arrhythmogenic right ventricular cardiomyopathy, which carries a much more sinister prognosis. Careful imaging of the right ventricle is therefore important to distinguish between these conditions in patients with ectopic beats arising from the right ventricle.

Even though some ventricular ectopics can precipitate fatal arrhythmias, routine treatment with anti-arrhythmic drugs has not been shown to decrease mortality. Some patients may be considerably troubled by symptoms caused by the ectopic beat, the compensatory pause or the following sinus beat (usually a feeling of 'extra' beats, 'missed' beats or 'heavy' beats) and will benefit from using an anti-arrhythmic agent. Where feasible, catheter ablation can be considered where symptoms are troublesome or there is a risk of malignant arrhythmias, and an ICD is also an option to provide protection from dangerous arrhythmias.

● Identifying the cardiac rhythm

If you have read through the first part of this chapter, you will now have a good idea of the range of normal and abnormal cardiac rhythms, and their causes and treatment, and will be in a good position to identify the cardiac rhythm in any ECG. If you have turned straight to this section, we strongly recommend that you spend some time going through the preceding pages before continuing any further.

In this section, we will teach you a routine to guide you towards the correct diagnosis of any rhythm disorder. Before doing this, we will repeat the warning with which we started this chapter.

SEEK HELP

If in doubt about a patient's cardiac rhythm, do not hesitate to seek the advice of a cardiologist.

We trust that the advice given here will be sufficient to keep you out of trouble when trying to identify the cardiac rhythm in an emergency. However, the recognition of some arrhythmias can be difficult, even for the specialist, and if you are at all uncertain about the diagnosis, it is important that you seek expert help at the earliest opportunity.

When you analyse the cardiac rhythm, always keep in mind the two questions that you are trying to answer:

- Where does the impulse arise from?
  - SA node
  - atria
  - AV junction
  - ventricles
- How is the impulse conducted?
  - normal conduction
  - accelerated conduction (e.g. WPW syndrome)
  - blocked conduction.

We will help you to narrow down the possible diagnoses with the following questions:

- How is the patient?
- Is ventricular activity present?
- What is the ventricular rate?

- Is the ventricular rhythm regular or irregular?
- Is the QRS complex width normal or broad?
- Is atrial activity present?
- How are atrial activity and ventricular activity related?

A similar approach to the ECG is used by the Resuscitation Council (UK) to train healthcare professionals in rhythm recognition. Attending an Advanced Life Support (ALS) course is an excellent way to improve your skills in cardiac rhythm recognition and, of course, in learning how to provide advanced life support. Contact details for the Resuscitation Council (UK) are provided in the chapter on further reading at the end of this book. If you live outside the UK, you should approach your local provider of ALS training for advice.

How is the patient?

Clinical context is all important in ECG interpretation, and you should not attempt to interpret an ECG rhythm without knowing the clinical context in which the ECG was recorded. Take the example of a rhythm strip that appears to show normal sinus rhythm. If it was recorded from a patient who is unconscious and pulseless, the rhythm will be pulseless electrical activity (PEA), not sinus rhythm. Similarly, the presence of artefact on an ECG can be misread as an arrhythmia unless the clinical context is known. To avoid these problems:

- If you are interpreting an ECG that someone else has recorded, always insist on knowing the clinical details of the patient and the reason why it was recorded.
- If you are recording an ECG that someone else will interpret later, always make a note of the clinical context at the top of the ECG to help with the interpretation (e.g. 'Patient complaining of rapid palpitations').

Is ventricular activity present?

Begin by looking at the ECG as a whole for the presence of electrical activity. If there is none, assess the patient (do they have a pulse?), the electrodes (has something become disconnected?) and the gain setting (is the gain setting on the monitor too low?).

If the patient is pulseless with no electrical activity evident on the ECG, they are in **asystole** and appropriate emergency action must be taken – see Chapter 17 for more details. Beware of diagnosing asystole in the presence of a completely flat ECG trace – there is usually some baseline drift present. A completely flat line usually means an electrode has become disconnected – check the electrodes (and, of course, the patient) carefully when making your diagnosis.

P waves may appear on their own (for a short time) after the onset of ventricular asystole. The presence of 'P waves only' on the ECG is important to recognize, as the patient may respond to emergency pacing manoeuvres such as percussion pacing, transcutaneous pacing or temporary transvenous pacing.

If QRS complexes are present, move on to the next question.

What is the ventricular rate?

Ventricular activity is represented on the ECG by QRS complexes. The two methods for determining the ventricular rate are discussed in Chapter 2. Once you have calculated the ventricular rate, you will be able to classify the rhythm as:

- bradycardia (<60 beats/min)
- normal (60–100 beats/min)
- tachycardia (>100 beats/min).

Is the ventricular rhythm regular or irregular?

Having determined the ventricular rate, you should determine its regularity. Look at the spacing between QRS complexes – is it the same throughout the rhythm strip? Irregularity can be subtle, so it is useful to measure out the distance between each QRS complex. One way to do this is to place a piece of paper alongside the rhythm strip and make a mark on it next to every

QRS complex. By moving the marked paper up and down along the rhythm strip, you can soon see if the gaps between the QRS complexes are the same or vary. Once you have assessed the regularity, you will be able to classify the ventricular rhythm as:

- regular (equal spacing between QRS complexes)
- irregular (variable spacing between QRS complexes).

Table 3.4 lists the causes of irregular cardiac rhythms.

Table 3.4 Irregular cardiac rhythms

- Atrial fibrillation
- Sinus arrhythmia
- Any supraventricular rhythm with intermittent AV block
- Ectopic beats

If the rhythm is irregular, it is helpful to try to characterize the degree of irregularity. **Atrial fibrillation**, for example, is a totally chaotic rhythm with no discernible pattern to the QRS complexes. **Sinus arrhythmia**, by comparison, shows a cyclical variation in ventricular rate that is not chaotic but has a clear periodicity to it, coinciding with the patient's breathing movements.

In **intermittent AV block**, if an impulse is blocked *en route* to the ventricles as a result of a conduction disturbance, the corresponding QRS complex will fail to appear where expected and the beat will be 'missed' (see Fig. 6.9, p. 122). This is discussed on page 119. The degree of irregularity will depend upon the nature of the conduction problem – the block of impulses may be predictable, in which case there will be a 'regular irregularity', or unpredictable.

Similarly, **ectopic beats** (Fig. 3.28) may occur in a predictable manner or unpredictably, giving rise to regular or irregular irregularities accordingly. In ventricular bigeminy, for example, a ventricular ectopic beat arises after each normal QRS complex, leading to a regular irregularity of the ventricular rhythm (see Fig. 3.27). Ectopic beats are discussed on page 61.

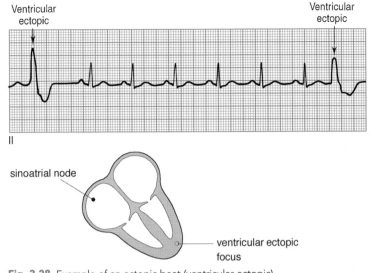

Fig. 3.28 Example of an ectopic beat (ventricular ectopic)

Key point: • ectopic beats appear earlier than expected

Is the QRS complex width normal or broad?

The width of the QRS complex can provide valuable clues about the origin of the cardiac rhythm. By answering this question, you will have narrowed down the origin of the impulse to one half of the heart. Ventricular rhythms are generated within the ventricular myocardium; supraventricular rhythms are generated anywhere up to (and including) the AV junction (Fig. 3.29).

Normally, the ventricles are depolarized via the His–Purkinje system, a network of rapidly conducting fibres that run throughout the ventricular myocardium. As a result, the ventricles are normally completely depolarized within 0.12 s, and the corresponding QRS complex on the ECG is less than 3 small squares wide.

However, if there is a problem with conduction within the ventricles, such as a block of part of the His–Purkinje system (as seen in left or right bundle branch block), depolarization has to spread directly from myocyte to myocyte instead. This takes

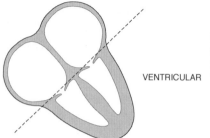

SUPRAVENTRICULAR

VENTRICULAR

Fig. 3.29 Supraventricular versus ventricular rhythms

Key point: • supraventricular applies to any structure above the ventricles (and electrically distinct from them)

longer, and so the QRS complex becomes wider than 3 small squares. This is also the case if the impulse has arisen within the ventricles (instead of coming via the AV node), as in the case of a ventricular ectopic beat or in VT. If an impulse does not pass through the AV node, it cannot use the His–Purkinje conduction system. Once again, it must travel from myocyte to myocyte, prolonging the process of depolarization.

This allows us to use the width of the QRS complex to try to determine how the ventricles were depolarized. If the QRS complex is narrow (<3 small squares), the ventricles must have been depolarized by an impulse that came through the AV node – the only way into the His–Purkinje system. The patient is then said to have a **supraventricular rhythm** (arising from above the ventricles).

If the QRS complex is broad (>3 small squares), there are two possible explanations:

1 The impulse may have arisen from within the ventricles and thus been unable to travel via the His–Purkinje system (**ventricular rhythm**).
2 The impulse may have arisen from above the ventricles but not been able to use all the His–Purkinje system because of a conduction problem (**supraventricular rhythm with aberrant conduction**).

This is summarized in Table 3.5.

Table 3.5 Broad-complex vs narrow-complex rhythms

	Broad complex	Narrow complex
Supraventricular rhythm with normal conduction	✗	✓
Supraventricular rhythm with aberrant conduction	✓	✗
Ventricular rhythm	✓	✗

Trying to distinguish between ventricular rhythms and supra-ventricular rhythms with aberrant conduction can be difficult, particularly if the patient is tachycardic and there is concern that the rhythm is VT. The distinction between VT and SVT is discussed specifically on page 74.

Is atrial activity present?

Atrial electrical activity can take several forms, which can be grouped into four categories:

● P waves (atrial depolarization)
● flutter waves (atrial flutter)
● fibrillation waves (AF)
● unclear activity.

The presence of **P waves** indicates atrial depolarization. This does not mean that the depolarization necessarily started at the SA node, however. P waves will appear during atrial depolarization regardless of where it originated – it is the *orientation* of the P waves that tells you where the depolarization originated (Chapter 5). Upright P waves in lead II suggest that atrial depolarization originated in or near the SA node. Inverted P waves suggest an origin closer to, or within, the AV node (Fig. 3.30).

Flutter waves are seen in atrial flutter at a rate of 300/min, creating a sawtooth baseline of atrial activity (see Fig. 3.11, p. 40). As discussed earlier, this can be made more readily apparent by manoeuvres that transiently block the AV node.

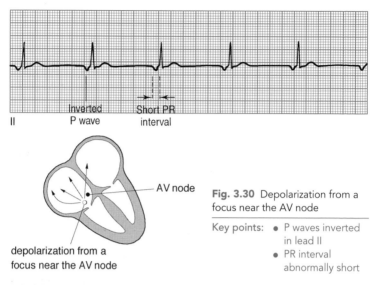

II   Inverted P wave   Short PR interval

AV node

depolarization from a focus near the AV node

Fig. 3.30 Depolarization from a focus near the AV node

Key points:
- P waves inverted in lead II
- PR interval abnormally short

Fibrillation waves are seen in AF and correspond to random, chaotic atrial impulses occurring at a rate of around 400–600/min (see Fig. 3.13). This leads to a chaotic, low-amplitude baseline of atrial activity.

The nature of the atrial activity may be **unclear**. This may be because P waves are 'hidden' within the QRS complexes, as is often the case during AV nodal re-entry tachycardia. In such cases atrial depolarization is taking place, but its electrical 'signature' on the ECG cannot easily be seen because the simultaneous, larger amplitude, QRS complex hides it. Atrial activity may also be absent in, for example, sinus arrest or SA block, in which case the atria may be electrically silent.

How are atrial activity and ventricular activity related?

Having examined the activity of the atria and of the ventricles, the final task is to determine how the two are related. Normally an impulse from the atria goes on to depolarize the ventricles, leading to a 1:1 relationship between P waves and QRS complexes. However, impulses from the atria may sometimes fail to reach the ventricles, or the ventricles may generate their own impulses independent of the atria.

If every QRS complex is associated with a P wave, this indicates that the atria and ventricles are being activated by a common source. This is usually, but not necessarily, the SA node (e.g. AV junctional rhythms will also depolarize both atria and ventricles).

If there are more P waves than QRS complexes, conduction between atria and ventricles is being either partly blocked (with only some impulses getting through) or completely blocked (with the ventricles having developed their own escape rhythm). An example is shown in Figure 3.31.

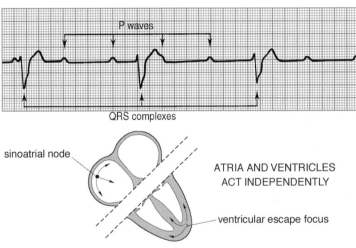

Fig. 3.31 Complete ('third-degree') AV block

Key points: • P wave rate is 75/min
• QRS rate is 33/min

More QRS complexes than P waves indicates AV dissociation (p. 125), with the ventricles operating independently of the atria and at a higher rate (Fig. 3.32).

Always bear in mind that the P wave may be difficult or even impossible to discern clearly. Therefore, it can be difficult to say conclusively that atrial activity is absent.

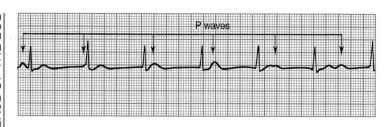

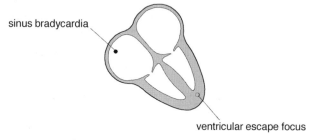

sinus bradycardia

ventricular escape focus

Fig. 3.32 AV dissociation

Key points:
- P wave rate 58/min
- QRS rate 65/min

Determining the cardiac rhythm

Using the seven questions above, you should be able to recognize most of the cardiac rhythms described in the first half of this chapter when you next encounter them. Always keep things simple and try to avoid getting side-tracked by unnecessary detail – the diagnosis will often be obvious once you have identified the key features of the ECG. There are a handful of rhythms that you should learn by rote so that you can recognize them without hesitation in an emergency – these are the **cardiac arrest rhythms** (VF, VT, asystole and pulseless electrical activity), which are discussed further in Chapter 17.

How do I distinguish between VT and SVT?

The distinction between VT and SVT with aberrant conduction is not always straightforward, as both can present with a broad-complex tachycardia on the ECG. The distinction is important, as the management of the two conditions is different (although in an emergency both VT and SVT usually respond to DC cardioversion). A good general rule is that *broad-complex tachycardia is always assumed to be VT unless proven otherwise*.

The clinical history may provide a pointer towards the correct diagnosis. A broad-complex tachycardia is more likely to be VT in elderly patients with a history of cardiac disease, and more likely to be SVT with aberrant conduction in young patients with no prior cardiac history. It should not be assumed that patients with VT will always be unwell – some patients tolerate VT remarkably well and can be virtually asymptomatic. Conversely, some patients tolerate SVT poorly.

A previous ECG may be helpful in determining whether aberrant conduction was present prior to the tachycardia, and whether the QRS morphology has changed. However, it is possible that aberrant conduction has developed in the period between the two ECGs, or that it only appears during the tachycardia. Broad complexes that display a typical left bundle branch block or right bundle branch block morphology (see Chapter 8) are more likely to be due to aberrant conduction; VT usually causes 'atypical' broad complexes that do not have the classic hallmarks of left or right bundle branch block.

A diagnostic feature of VT is the presence of **independent atrial activity**, although it is found in fewer than half of cases. Independent atrial activity is indicated by:

- independent P wave activity
- fusion beats
- capture beats.

Independent P wave activity is shown by the presence of P waves occurring at a slower rate than the QRS complexes and bearing no relation to them (Fig. 3.33). It can, however, be difficult or even impossible to discern P waves during VT.

Fusion beats appear when the ventricles are activated by an atrial impulse and a ventricular impulse arriving simultaneously (Fig. 3.34).

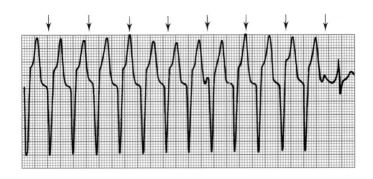

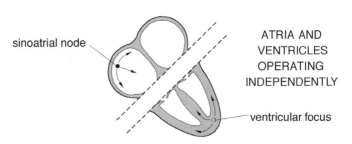

Fig. 3.33 Independent P wave activity

Key points:
- broad-complex tachycardia (VT)
- arrows show independent P waves deforming the QRS complexes
- last beat is a capture beat

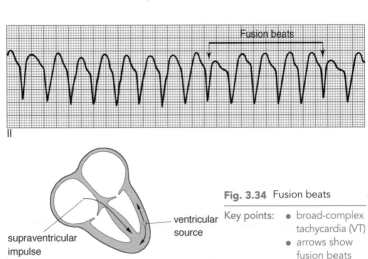

II

Fusion beats

Fig. 3.34 Fusion beats

Key points:
- broad-complex tachycardia (VT)
- arrows show fusion beats

Capture beats occur when an atrial impulse manages to 'capture' the ventricles for a beat, causing a normal QRS complex, which may be preceded by a normal P wave (Fig. 3.35).

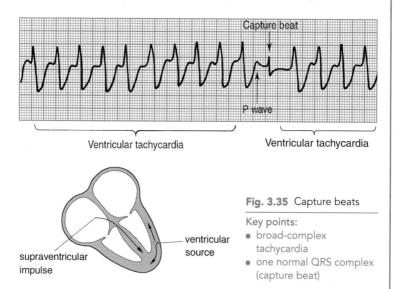

Ventricular tachycardia   Ventricular tachycardia

Fig. 3.35 Capture beats

Key points:
- broad-complex tachycardia
- one normal QRS complex (capture beat)

● Supraventricular tachycardia

The term 'supraventricular tachycardia' is frequently misused and this leads to misunderstanding. Literally, it refers to any heart rate over 100 beats/min (tachycardia) that originates above the ventricles (supraventricular). It encompasses many different arrhythmias, including sinus tachycardia, AF, atrial tachycardia and AV re-entry tachycardias. This is the meaning of SVT that has been used in this book. Some people use the term SVT to refer specifically to AV nodal re-entry tachycardias. We recommend that you identify all arrhythmias as specifically as possible, and reserve SVT as a general term for tachycardias that originate above the ventricles.

Other clues that suggest that a broad-complex tachycardia is due to VT are:

- QRS duration >0.14 s (3.5 small squares)
- concordance (same QRS direction) in leads V_1–V_6
- a shift in QRS axis of 40° or more (left or right).

If the rhythm slows or terminates with manoeuvres that slow or block conduction in the AV node, it is likely to be supraventricular with aberrant conduction.

Summary

When assessing the cardiac rhythm, consider the following:

- SA nodal rhythms
  - sinus rhythm
  - sinus bradycardia
  - sinus tachycardia
  - sinus arrhythmia
  - sick sinus syndrome
- Atrial rhythms
  - atrial tachycardia
  - atrial flutter
  - AF
- AV rhythms
- AV re-entry tachycardias
- Ventricular rhythms
  - VT
  - accelerated idioventricular rhythm
  - torsades de pointes (polymorphic VT)
  - VF
- Conduction disturbances
- Escape rhythms
- Ectopic beats.

To identify the rhythm, ask yourself the following questions:

1. Where does the impulse arise from?

- SA node
- Atria
- AV junction
- Ventricles.

2. How is the impulse conducted?

- Normal conduction
- Accelerated conduction (e.g. WPW syndrome)
- Blocked conduction.

The axis **4**

Working out the cardiac axis causes more confusion than almost any other aspect of ECG assessment. This should not really be the case, as there is no mystery to the cardiac axis and it is usually straightforward to assess. Indeed, deciding whether the cardiac axis is normal can be summarized in one rule.

● A quick rule for assessing the axis
  If the QRS complexes are predominantly positive in leads I and II, the cardiac axis is normal.

If you are confident about assessing the axis, you can go straight to the second half of this chapter, where we explain the causes of an abnormal axis. If not, read through the first half of the chapter, where we explain in straightforward terms what the axis represents and how it can be measured.

● Understanding and measuring the cardiac axis

What does the axis mean?

As we explained in Chapter 1, the flow of electrical current through the heart is fairly uniform, as it normally passes along a well-defined pathway (Fig. 4.1).

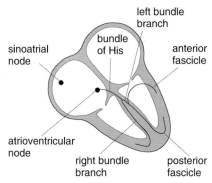

Fig. 4.1 The flow of electrical impulses through the heart

Key points: • impulses originate in the sinoatrial node
• impulses reach the ventricles via the atrioventricular node

In simple terms, the cardiac axis is an indicator of the general direction that the wave of depolarization takes as it flows through the heart. If you think just about the general direction of electrical current as it flows through the ventricles, it starts at the 'top right hand corner' and flows towards the 'bottom left hand corner' (Fig. 4.2).

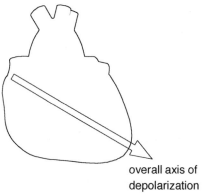

overall axis of
depolarization

Fig. 4.2 The general direction of flow of electrical current through the heart

Key points: • flow starts at the 'top right hand corner'
• flow is towards the 'bottom left hand corner'

What measurement is used for the axis?

When describing the axis, a more precise terminology is required. The axis is therefore conventionally referred to as the angle, measured in degrees, of the direction of electrical current flowing through the heart.

The reference, or zero, point is taken as a horizontal line 'looking' at the heart from the left (Fig. 4.3). For a direction of flow directed below the line, the angle is expressed as a positive number; above the line, as a negative number (Fig. 4.4). Thus, the cardiac axis can be either +1° to +180°, or −1° to −180°.

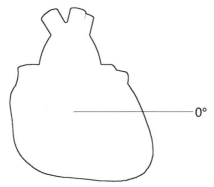

Fig. 4.3 The reference (or 'zero') point for axis measurements

Key points:
- the zero point is a horizontal line looking at the heart from the left
- this is the same as the viewpoint of lead I
- all axis measurements are made relative to this line

You will remember from Chapter 1 that the six limb leads look at the heart sideways from six different viewpoints. The same reference system can be used to describe the angle from which each lead looks at the heart (Fig. 4.5). The limb leads and their angles are listed in Table 4.1.

Make an effort to remember the viewpoint of each limb lead now, before reading any further. Once you have grasped the concept of each limb lead having a different angle of view of the heart, understanding the cardiac axis will be easy.

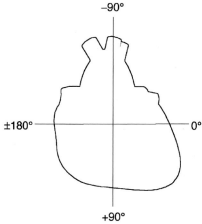

Fig. 4.4 The range of angles of the cardiac axis

Key points:
- anticlockwise measurements are negative
- clockwise measurements are positive
- all measurements are relative to the zero line

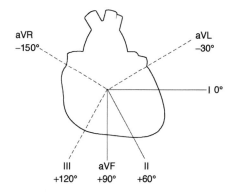

Fig. 4.5 Viewpoints of the six limb leads

Key point:
- each lead looks at the heart from a different angle

Table 4.1 Limb leads and angles of view

Limb lead	Angle at which it views the heart
I	0°
II	+60°
III	+120°
aVR	−150°
aVL	−30°
aVF	+90°

How do I use the limb leads to work out the axis?

The information from the limb leads is used to work out the cardiac axis. Simply remember three principles, all of which we have covered already:

- The axis is the general direction of electrical flow through the heart.
- Each of the limb leads records this electrical flow from a different viewpoint of the heart.
- Electrical flow towards a lead causes a positive deflection, and flow away from a lead causes a negative deflection.

The last rule means that if current flows at right angles to a lead, the ECG complex generated will be isoelectric, that is the positive and negative deflections cancel each other out. This is illustrated in Figure 4.6.

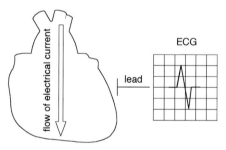

Fig. 4.6 An isoelectric ECG complex

Key point: • current flow at right angles to a lead causes an isoelectric complex

Using these principles, consider how lead II records ventricular depolarization. From its point of view, the flow of current in the ventricles is entirely towards it and the QRS complex is entirely positive (Fig. 4.7). Lead aVL, however, will see the same current at right angles to itself and record an isoelectric QRS complex (Fig. 4.8). Any lead looking from a viewpoint between leads II and aVL will record a complex that becomes increasingly positive the closer i is to lead II (Fig. 4.9).

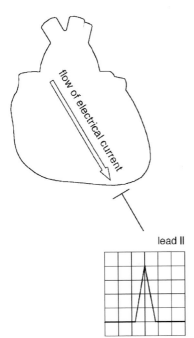

Fig. 4.7 The QRS complex is entirely positive in lead II

Key points:
- flow towards a lead causes a positive deflection
- current flow in the ventricles is towards lead II

lead II

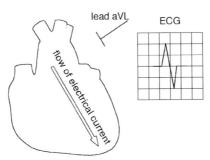

Fig. 4.8 The QRS complex is isoelectric in lead aVL

Key points:
- flow at right angles to a lead causes an isoelectric complex
- current flow in the ventricles is at right angles to lead aVL

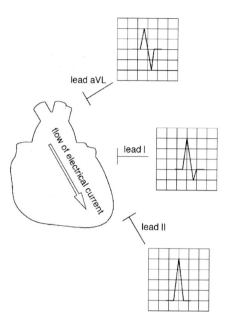

Fig. 4.9 The QRS complex is predominantly positive in lead I

Key point: • lead I lies between leads II and aVL

It should now be fairly clear that you can work out the cardiac axis by examining whether the QRS complexes in the limb leads are predominantly positive or negative.

There are two ways of determining the cardiac axis: one is quick and approximate, the other is precise but detailed.

● What is a 'normal' axis?

Unfortunately, there is no universal agreement on what is a normal axis. For the purposes of this book, we consider a normal axis to be anything between −30° and +90°, although we should mention that some cardiologists accept anything up to +120° as normal. This is because there is no definitive dividing line between normality and abnormality. The most sensible approach is to consider that the likelihood of a patient having an underlying abnormality increases as the axis increases from +90° to +120°.

A quick way to work out the cardiac axis

This technique enables you to decide within seconds whether the axis is normal or abnormal. To decide if the axis is normal, you need only look at two of the limb leads: I and II.

If the QRS complex in **lead I** is predominantly positive, this indicates that the axis lies anywhere between −90° and +90° (Fig. 4.10). An axis at *exactly* −90° or +90° would cause a precisely isoelectric QRS complex in lead I. Thus, a predominantly positive QRS complex in lead I rules out right axis deviation (an axis beyond +90°), but does not exclude left axis deviation (an axis beyond −30°).

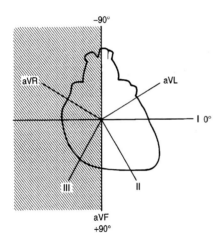

Fig. 4.10 A predominantly positive QRS in lead I puts the axis between −90° and +90°

Key point: • a predominantly positive QRS in lead I excludes right axis deviation

If the QRS complex in **lead II** is predominantly positive, this indicates that the axis lies anywhere between −30° and +150° (Fig. 4.11). An axis at *exactly* −30° or +150° would cause a precisely isoelectric QRS complex in lead II. Thus, a predominantly positive QRS complex in lead II rules out left axis deviation (an axis beyond −30°), but does not exclude right axis deviation (an axis beyond +90°).

However, by looking at whether the QRS complex is positive or negative in both these leads, it is possible to say immediately

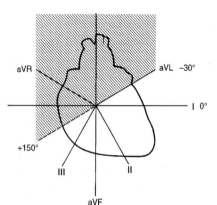

Fig. 4.11 A predominantly positive QRS in lead II puts the axis between −30° and +150°

Key point: ● a predominantly positive QRS in lead II excludes left axis deviation

whether the axis is normal, or whether there is left or right axis deviation:

● A predominantly positive QRS complex in both leads I and II means the **axis is normal**.
● A predominantly positive QRS complex in lead I and a predominantly negative QRS complex in lead II mean there is **left axis deviation**.
● A predominantly negative QRS complex in lead I and a predominantly positive QRS complex in lead II mean there is **right axis deviation**.

These rules are summarized in Table 4.2.

Table 4.2 Working out the cardiac axis

Lead I	Lead II	Cardiac axis
Positive QRS	Positive QRS	Normal axis
Positive QRS	Negative QRS	Left axis deviation
Negative QRS	Positive QRS	Right axis deviation

When you assess the cardiac axis you should therefore ask the following questions:

● Is there left axis deviation?
● Is there right axis deviation?

The causes of these abnormalities, with guidance on their management, are discussed in the second half of this chapter.

A more precise way to calculate the cardiac axis

For most practical purposes, it is not necessary to determine precisely the axis of the heart – it is sufficient to know simply whether the axis is normal or abnormal. Calculating the axis precisely is not difficult but does take a little time, and this section explains how.

The method relies on the use of vectors and knowledge of how to calculate angles in right-angled triangles. Begin by finding two leads that look at the heart at right angles to each other, for example leads I and aVF (Fig. 4.12).

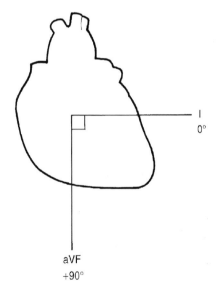

Fig. 4.12 Leads I and aVF

Key point: • leads I and aVF are at right angles to each other

Look at the QRS complexes in the leads in Figure 4.13 and work out their overall sizes and polarities by subtracting the depth of the S wave from the height of the R wave. The polarity (positive or negative) tells you whether the impulse is moving towards or away from the lead. The overall size tells you how much of the electricity is flowing in that direction. Using this information, you can construct a vector diagram (Fig. 4.14).

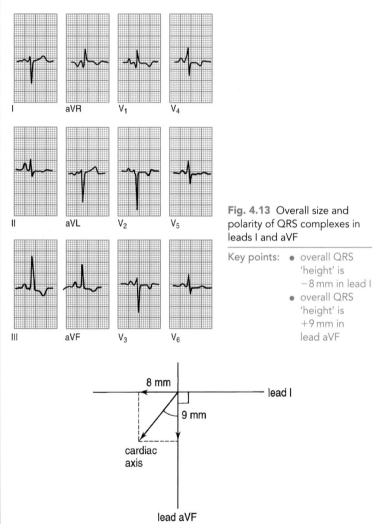

I	aVR	V$_1$	V$_4$
II	aVL	V$_2$	V$_5$
III	aVF	V$_3$	V$_6$

Fig. 4.13 Overall size and polarity of QRS complexes in leads I and aVF

Key points:
- overall QRS 'height' is −8 mm in lead I
- overall QRS 'height' is +9 mm in lead aVF

8 mm

9 mm

lead I

cardiac axis

lead aVF

Fig. 4.14 Constructing a vector diagram

Key points:
- draw arrows to represent the QRS 'heights' from Figure 4.13
- the cardiac axis lies between the arrows
- use sine, cosine or tangent to work out the exact angle of the axis

Thus, by combining the information from the two leads, you can use a pocket calculator to work out the angle at which the current is flowing (i.e. the cardiac axis).

> ● Remember
>   • Sine of an angle = opposite edge/hypotenuse
>   • Cosine of an angle = adjacent edge/hypotenuse
>   • Tangent of an angle = opposite edge/adjacent edge

Thus, we finally arrive at an angle in degrees (Fig. 4.15). Do not forget that the cardiac axis is measured relative to lead I, and to add or subtract units of 90° accordingly. The axis in the patient in Figure 4.12 is therefore +132°, and he or she has (by our definition) right axis deviation. We recommend that you practise this technique to become fully familiar with it.

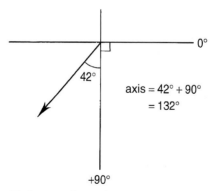

Fig. 4.15 Working out the cardiac axis

Key point: ● do not forget to add or subtract units of 90° according to which quadrant the axis lies in

- ● P and T wave axes
  So far, we have concentrated on the axis of depolarization as it flows through the ventricles, and this is generally referred to as the cardiac axis. However, it is also
  possible to work out an axis for atrial depolarization (by
  applying the vector analysis we have described to
  P waves) and for ventricular repolarization (using T waves).
  These measurements are seldom necessary, except
  where a more detailed analysis of the ECG is required.

● Is there left axis deviation?

Left axis deviation is present when the cardiac axis lies beyond
−30°. This sometimes occurs in normal individuals, but more
often indicates one of the following:

- left anterior hemiblock
- Wolff–Parkinson–White (WPW) syndrome
- inferior myocardial infarction
- ventricular tachycardia.

These are discussed below.

Left ventricular hypertrophy can cause left axis deviation but
not as a result of increased muscle mass (unlike right ventricular hypertrophy). Instead, it results from left anterior hemiblock caused by fibrosis. Contrary to some textbooks, neither
obesity nor pregnancy causes left axis deviation (although
obesity can cause a *leftward shift* with the axis staying within
normal limits).

Left anterior hemiblock

In Chapter 1, we describe how electrical impulses are conducted within the interventricular septum in the left and right
bundle branches, and that the left bundle branch divides
into anterior and posterior fascicles (Fig. 4.1, p. 81). Either

(or both) of these fascicles can be blocked. Block of the left anterior fascicle is called left anterior hemiblock, and is the commonest cause of left axis deviation (Fig. 4.16).

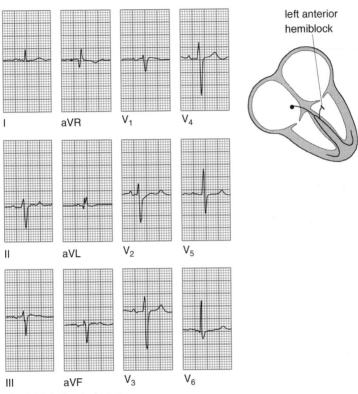

Fig. 4.16 Left axis deviation

Key points:
- QRS is positive in lead I and negative in lead II
- the cardiac axis is $-48°$

Left anterior hemiblock can occur as a result of fibrosis of the conducting system (of any cause) or from myocardial infarction. On its own, it is not thought to carry any prognostic significance. However, left anterior hemiblock in combination with right bundle branch block (p. 148) means that two of the three main conducting pathways to the ventricles are blocked. This is termed **bifascicular block** (Fig. 4.17).

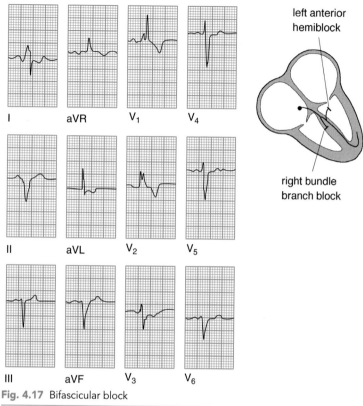

left anterior
hemiblock

right bundle
branch block

Fig. 4.17 Bifascicular block

Key point: • left axis deviation (cardiac axis is −82°)
            • right bundle branch block

Block of the conducting pathways can occur in any combination. A block of both fascicles is the equivalent of left bundle branch block. Block of the right bundle branch and either fascicle is bifascicular block. If bifascicular block is combined with first-degree AV block (long PR interval), this is called **trifascicular block** (Fig. 4.18). Block of the right bundle branch and both fascicles leaves no route for impulses to reach the ventricles, and this is the equivalent of third-degree ('complete') AV block.

Bifascicular block in a patient with syncopal episodes is often sufficient indication for a permanent pacemaker, even if higher

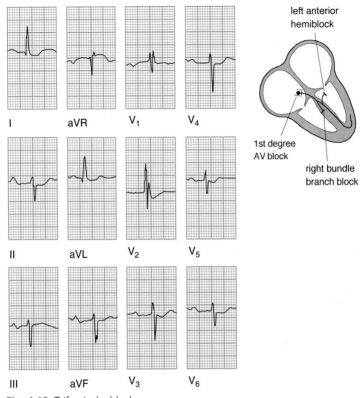

left anterior
hemiblock

1st degree
AV block

right bundle
branch block

I aVR V₁ V₄

II aVL V₂ V₅

III aVF V₃ V₆

Fig. 4.18 Trifascicular block

Key points: • left axis deviation (cardiac axis is −38°)
             • right bundle branch block
             • first-degree AV block (PR interval is 0.32 s)

degrees of block have not been documented. You should therefore refer these patients to a cardiologist. *Asymptomatic* bifascicular block, or even trifascicular block, is not necessarily an
indication for pacing – discuss with a cardiologist.

SEEK HELP

Bifascicular block with syncope usually requires pacing.
Referral to a cardiologist is recommended.

Wolff–Parkinson–White syndrome

Patients with Wolff–Parkinson–White (WPW) syndrome have an accessory pathway that bypasses the atrioventricular node and bundle of His to connect the atria directly to the ventricles. If this pathway lies between the atria and ventricles on the right side of the heart, patients may have left axis deviation in addition to the other ECG appearances of WPW syndrome (discussed on p. 114).

Inferior myocardial infarction

Left axis deviation may be a feature of myocardial infarction affecting the inferior aspect of the heart (the cardiac axis is directed away from infarcted areas). The diagnosis will usually be apparent from the presentation and other ECG findings. For more information on the diagnosis and treatment of acute myocardial infarction, see Chapter 9.

Ventricular tachycardia (with a focus in the left ventricle apex)

When ventricular tachycardia arises from a focus in the left ventricle apex, the wave of depolarization spreads out through the rest of the myocardium from that point, resulting in left axis deviation. The diagnosis and treatment of ventricular tachycardia are discussed on page 53.

● Is there right axis deviation?

Right axis deviation is present when the cardiac axis lies beyond +90°. This sometimes occurs in normal individuals, but more often indicates one of the following:

- right ventricular hypertrophy
- WPW syndrome
- anterolateral myocardial infarction
- dextrocardia
- left posterior hemiblock.

These are discussed below.

Right ventricular hypertrophy

Right ventricular hypertrophy is the commonest cause of right axis deviation (Fig. 4.19). Other ECG evidence of right ventricular hypertrophy includes:

- dominant R wave in lead V_1
- deep S waves in leads V_5 and V_6
- right bundle branch block.

For more information on the causes of right ventricular hypertrophy, turn to page 139.

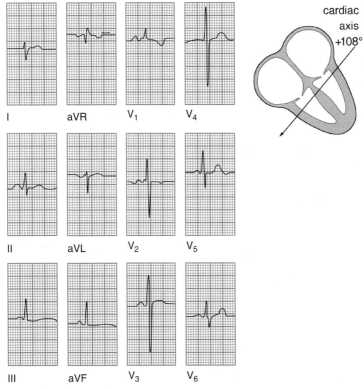

Fig. 4.19 Right axis deviation

Key points:
- QRS is negative in lead I and positive in lead II
- right ventricular hypertrophy is present
- cardiac axis is +108°

Wolff–Parkinson–White syndrome

As with right-sided accessory pathways and left axis deviation, patients with WPW syndrome who have a left-sided accessory pathway may have right axis deviation in addition to the other ECG appearances of WPW syndrome. WPW syndrome is discussed in more detail on page 114.

Anterolateral myocardial infarction

The cardiac axis is directed away from infarcted areas. Thus, right axis deviation may be a feature of anterolateral myocardial infarction. The diagnosis will usually be apparent from the presentation and other ECG findings. For more information on the diagnosis and treatment of acute myocardial infarction, see Chapter 9.

Dextrocardia

Right axis deviation is a feature of dextrocardia (in which the heart lies on the right side of the chest instead of the left), but the most obvious abnormality is that all the chest leads have 'right ventricular' QRS complexes (see Fig. 8.5, p. 143). Dextrocardia is discussed in more detail on page 142.

Left posterior hemiblock

Unlike left anterior hemiblock, left posterior hemiblock is extremely rare. It is identified in approximately only 1 in 10 000 ECGs. It is therefore extremely important that if you identify right axis deviation on an ECG, you rule out other causes (in particular, right ventricular hypertrophy) before diagnosing left posterior hemiblock. The causes and management of left posterior hemiblock are the same as for left anterior hemiblock (p. 92).

Summary

To assess the cardiac axis, ask the following questions:

1. Is there left axis deviation?

If 'yes', consider:

- left anterior hemiblock
- WPW syndrome
- inferior myocardial infarction
- ventricular tachycardia (with left ventricular apical focus).

2. Is there right axis deviation?

If 'yes', consider:

- right ventricular hypertrophy
- WPW syndrome
- anterolateral myocardial infarction
- dextrocardia
- left posterior hemiblock.

The P wave

After determining the heart rate, rhythm and axis, you should examine each wave of the ECG in turn, beginning with the P wave. You may already have noticed abnormal P waves while assessing the cardiac rhythm, but in this chapter we tell you how to examine the P wave in more detail and what abnormalities to look out for.

As you examine the P wave in each lead, the questions to ask are:

- Are any P waves absent?
- Are any P waves inverted?
- Are any P waves too tall?
- Are any P waves too wide?

- The origin of the P wave
  You will recall from Chapter 1 that the P wave represents atrial depolarization. It does not, as some people mistakenly believe, represent sinoatrial (SA) node depolarization; it is possible to have P waves without SA node depolarization (e.g. atrial ectopics) or SA node depolarization without P waves (SA block).

● Are any P waves absent?

The SA node is normally a regular and dependable natural pacemaker. Atrial depolarization (and thus P wave formation) is therefore normally so regular that it is easy to predict when the next P wave is going to appear (Fig. 5.1).

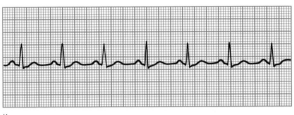

II

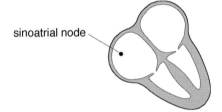

sinoatrial node

Fig. 5.1 Sinus rhythm

Key points: ● regular P waves
● it is easy to predict when the next P wave will appear

The only normal circumstance in which the P wave rate is variable is sinus arrhythmia, which is usually only seen in patients below the age of 40 years. Sinus arrhythmia is discussed on page 34.

In this section, we tell you what diagnoses to consider if you find that P waves are absent. By this, we mean that they can be either:

● completely absent (no P waves on the whole ECG), or
● intermittently absent (some P waves do not appear where expected).

P waves are completely absent

There are two reasons why P waves may be absent from the ECG. The first is that there is no coordinated atrial depolarization so that P waves are not being formed. The second is that P waves *are* present, but are just not obvious.

A lack of coordinated atrial depolarization occurs in atrial fibrillation, and this is the commonest reason for P waves to be truly absent from the ECG (Fig. 5.2). Instead of P waves, the chaotic atrial activity produces low-amplitude oscillations (fibrillation or 'f' waves) on the ECG. Atrial fibrillation can be recognized by the absence of P waves and the erratic formation of QRS complexes. Atrial fibrillation is discussed on page 42.

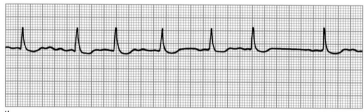

II

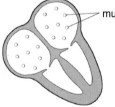

multiple atrial foci

Fig. 5.2 Atrial fibrillation

Key points: • absent P waves
 • erratic ('irregularly irregular') QRS rhythm

P waves will also be completely absent if there is a prolonged period of sinus arrest or sinoatrial block (Fig. 5.3). In these conditions, atrial activation does not occur because the SA node either fails to depolarize (sinus arrest) or fails to transmit the depolarization to the atria (SA block). Either condition *can* cause ventricular asystole, but more commonly an escape rhythm takes over (p. 59). See page 35 for more information on sinus arrest and SA block.

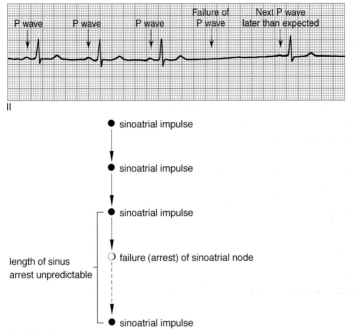

Fig. 5.3 Sinus arrest

Key points: • failure of P wave to appear when predicted
• the next P wave appears later than expected
• the sinoatrial 'clock' has therefore reset

Absent P waves are also one of the possible ECG manifest-ations of hyperkalaemia (p. 187). If this is a possibility, look for associated ECG abnormalities and check the patient's plasma potassium level urgently.

It is very common for P waves to be present but not immedi-ately obvious. Search the ECG carefully for evidence of P waves before concluding that they are absent, as P waves will often be hidden by any rapid tachycardia. In normal sinus rhythm the P waves are usually best seen in leads II and V_1, and so these leads should be examined particularly closely. Figure 5.4 shows an atrioventricular (AV) junctional tachycardia with a heart rate of 130 beats/min. At first glance, the P waves appear to be

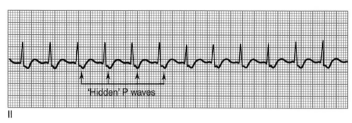

II

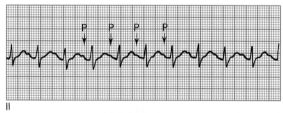

sinoatrial node

Fig. 5.4 AV junctional tachycardia

Key points:
- heart rate is 130 beats/min
- narrow QRS complexes
- P waves 'hidden' within the ST segments

absent. On closer inspection, they can just be seen buried within the ST segments.

Even in sinus tachycardia, at high heart rates the P waves may start to overlap with the T waves of the previous beats, making them hard to identify (Fig. 5.5).

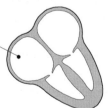

II

Fig. 5.5 Sinus tachycardia

Key points:
- heart rate is 130 beats/min
- narrow QRS complexes
- P waves 'hidden' within the previous T waves

sinoatrial node

At very high atrial rates, such as in atrial flutter, P waves may not be apparent because they become distorted. In atrial flutter, the atria usually depolarize around 300 times/min. The P waves generated by this rapid activity are called flutter waves, and have a 'sawtooth' appearance. Atrial flutter is discussed on page 39.

In ventricular tachycardia, retrograde (backward) conduction up through the AV node may cause each QRS complex to be *followed* by a P wave which may not be immediately obvious and which also, incidentally, will be inverted. Even more importantly, *independent* atrial activity can occur during ventricular tachycardia, and the P waves can be buried anywhere within the QRS complexes (see Fig. 3.33, p. 76). Evidence of independent atrial activity is a very useful clue in the differentiation of ventricular and supraventricular tachycardias.

More information about all of these cardiac rhythms can be found in Chapter 3.

P waves are intermittently absent

The SA node is usually an extremely reliable natural pacemaker. The occasional absence of a P wave on an ECG indicates that the SA node has either failed to generate an impulse (sinus arrest) or failed to conduct the impulse to the surrounding atrial tissue (SA block).

For examples of both these conditions, together with guidance on how to distinguish them, see page 35.

● Are any P waves inverted?

The P wave is usually upright in all leads except aVR, which 'looks' at the atria from roughly the patient's right shoulder and so detects the wave of atrial depolarization moving away from it (see Fig. 1.8, p. 7). The P wave may sometimes be inverted in lead V_1 also, although it is more usually biphasic in that lead (Fig. 5.6).

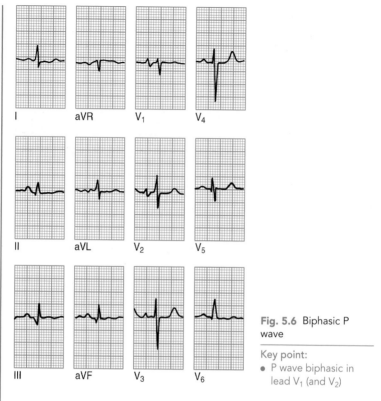

Fig. 5.6 Biphasic P wave

Key point:
- P wave biphasic in lead V_1 (and V_2)

Whenever you see an inverted P wave, ask yourself:

- Were the electrodes correctly positioned?

Abnormal P wave inversion can indicate either of the following:

- dextrocardia
- abnormal atrial depolarization.

Dextrocardia is discussed on page 142. Abnormal atrial depolarization is explained below.

Abnormal atrial depolarization

The wave of depolarization normally spreads through the atria from the SA node to the AV node. If atrial depolarization is initiated from within, near or through the AV node, the wave will travel in the opposite (retrograde) direction through the atria. From the 'viewpoints' of most of the ECG leads, this wave will be moving *away from* rather than towards them, and *inverted* P waves will be produced (Fig. 5.7).

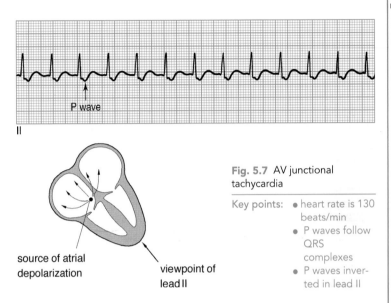

II

source of atrial depolarization

viewpoint of lead II

Fig. 5.7 AV junctional tachycardia

Key points:
- heart rate is 130 beats/min
- P waves follow QRS complexes
- P waves inverted in lead II

Many abnormal sources of atrial activation can thus cause retrograde depolarization and inverted P waves, including:

- atrial ectopics
- AV junctional rhythms
- ventricular tachycardia (retrogradely conducted)
- ventricular ectopics (retrogradely conducted).

A discussion of how to identify and manage all of these rhythms can be found in Chapter 3.

● Are any P waves too tall?

Normal P waves are usually less than 0.25 mV (2.5 small squares) in amplitude. Tall, peaked P waves indicate right atrial enlargement. The abnormality is sometimes referred to as 'P pulmonale', because right atrial enlargement is often secondary to pulmonary disorders. An example is shown in Figure 5.8.

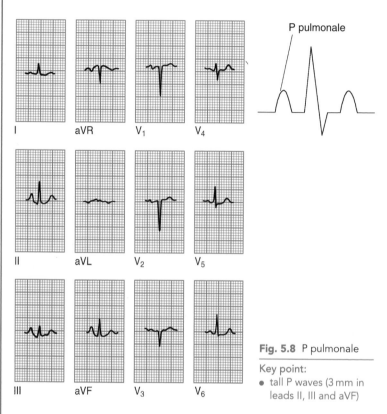

I aVR V₁ V₄

II aVL V₂ V₅

III aVF V₃ V₆

P pulmonale

Fig. 5.8 P pulmonale

Key point:
- tall P waves (3 mm in leads II, III and aVF)

If the P waves appear unusually tall, assess your patient for any of the causes of right atrial enlargement (Table 5.1).

Abnormally tall P waves should draw attention to the possibility of an underlying disorder that may require further

Table 5.1 Causes of right atrial enlargement

- Primary pulmonary hypertension
- Secondary pulmonary hypertension
  - chronic bronchitis
  - emphysema
  - massive pulmonary embolism
- Pulmonary stenosis
- Tricuspid stenosis

investigation. In addition to a thorough patient history and examination, a chest radiograph (to assess cardiac dimensions and lung fields) and an echocardiogram (to assess valvular disorders and estimate pulmonary artery pressure) may be helpful.

● Are any P waves too wide?

Normal P waves are usually less than 0.12 s (3 small squares) in duration. Minor notching of the P wave ('bifid' P wave) is not uncommon, indicating a mild degree of asynchrony between right and left atrial depolarization, but any broadening of the P wave with a notch greater than 0.1 mV (1 small square) in depth should arouse suspicion of left atrial enlargement. This is usually a result of mitral valve disease, and consequently these broad, bifid P waves are known as 'P mitrale' (Fig. 5.9).

The P wave becomes broad because the enlarged left atrium takes longer than normal to depolarize. As with P pulmonale, P mitrale does not require treatment in its own right, but should alert you to a possible underlying problem. This is often mitral valve disease, but left atrial enlargement can also accompany left ventricular hypertrophy (e.g. secondary to hypertension, aortic valve disease and hypertrophic cardiomyopathy). A chest X-ray and an echocardiogram may be helpful following a patient history and examination.

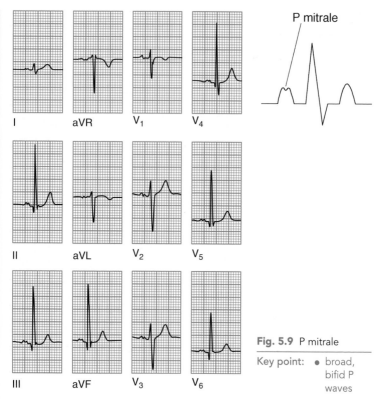

I aVR V₁ V₄
II aVL V₂ V₅
III aVF V₃ V₆

P mitrale

Fig. 5.9 P mitrale

Key point: • broad, bifid P waves

Summary

To assess the P wave, ask the following questions:

1. Are any P waves absent?

If 'yes', consider:

- P waves are completely absent
  - sinus arrest or SA block (prolonged)
  - hyperkalaemia
- P waves are present but not obvious
- P waves are intermittently absent
  - sinus arrest or SA block (intermittent).

2. Are any P waves inverted?

If 'yes', consider:

- electrode misplacement
- dextrocardia
- retrograde atrial depolarization.

3. Are any P waves too tall?

If 'yes', consider:
- right atrial enlargement.

4. Are any P waves too wide?

If 'yes', consider:
- left atrial enlargement.

The PR interval **6**

Once the sinus node has generated an electrical stimulus, this must be transmitted through the atria, atrioventricular (AV) node and bundle of His to reach the ventricles and bring about cardiac contraction. The time delay while this occurs is mainly taken up by the passage of the electrical impulse through the AV node, which acts as a regulator of conduction. This corresponds to the PR interval on the ECG (Fig. 6.1).

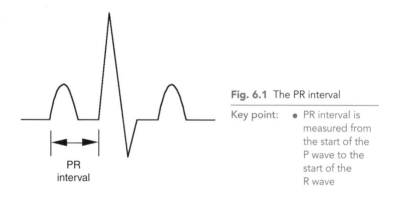

Fig. 6.1 The PR interval

Key point:
- PR interval is measured from the start of the P wave to the start of the R wave

The PR interval has precise time limits. In health, this interval is:

- no less than 0.12 s (3 small squares) long
- no more than 0.2 s (5 small squares) long
- consistent in length.

Make sure you check the duration of as many consecutive PR intervals as you can and ask the following questions:

- Is the PR interval less than 0.12 s long?
- Is the PR interval more than 0.2 s long?
- Does the PR interval vary or can it not be measured?

This chapter will help you to answer these questions and to reach a diagnosis if you find any abnormalities.

● Is the PR interval less than 0.12 s long?

A PR interval of less than 0.12 s (3 small squares) indicates that the usual delay to conduction between the atria and the ventricles, imposed by the AV junction, has not occurred. This happens if depolarization *originates* in the AV junction, so that it travels up to the atria and down to the ventricles simultaneously, or if it originates as normal in the sinus node but bypasses the AV junction via an *additional faster-conducting pathway.*

A short PR interval should therefore prompt you to think of:

- AV nodal rhythm
- Wolff–Parkinson–White (WPW) syndrome
- Lown–Ganong–Levine (LGL) syndrome.

Details of how to recognize and manage each of these are given below.

AV nodal rhythm

If depolarization is initiated from within the AV node, the wave of atrial depolarization will travel backwards through the atria at the same time as setting off forwards through the AV node towards the ventricles. Thus, the time delay between atrial depolarization (the P wave) and ventricular depolarization (the QRS complex) will be reduced (Fig. 6.2).

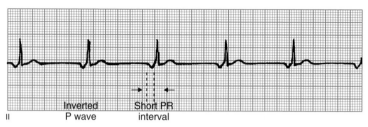

Fig. 6.2 Depolarization from a focus in the AV node

Key points:
- P waves inverted in lead II
- PR interval abnormally short

Any source of depolarization within the AV node can therefore cause a short PR interval, including:

- AV nodal escape rhythms
- AV ectopics
- AV re-entry tachycardia.

A discussion of how to identify and manage all of these rhythms can be found in Chapter 3. Atrial ectopics arising near to the AV node will also have a shorter PR interval than normal sinus beats, but it will rarely be less than 0.12 s long.

Wolff–Parkinson–White syndrome

In most people, conduction of electricity through the heart follows just one distinct path from atria to ventricles, namely via the AV node, bundle of His and Purkinje fibres. Some people have an additional connection between the atria and the ventricles – this is WPW syndrome (Fig. 6.3).

The accessory pathway (called the bundle of Kent) conducts more quickly than the AV node, so the wave of depolarization reaches the ventricles more quickly than usual and thus the

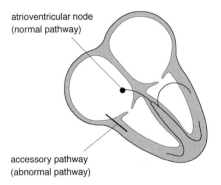

atrioventricular node
(normal pathway)

accessory pathway
(abnormal pathway)

Fig. 6.3 Wolff–Parkinson–White syndrome

Key point: ● accessory pathway between atria and ventricles

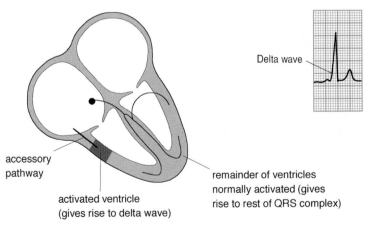

PR interval is short. The region of ventricle activated via the accessory pathway slowly depolarizes, giving rise to a **delta wave** – the first part of the QRS complex (Fig. 6.4). Shortly afterwards, the rest of the ventricular muscle is depolarized rapidly with the arrival of the normally conducted wave of depolarization via the AV node.

Delta wave

accessory pathway

activated ventricle
(gives rise to delta wave)

remainder of ventricles normally activated (gives rise to rest of QRS complex)

Fig. 6.4 Delta wave

Key point: ● the slurred upstroke of the QRS complex is the delta wave

Figure 6.5 shows a 12-lead ECG recorded from a patient with WPW syndrome.

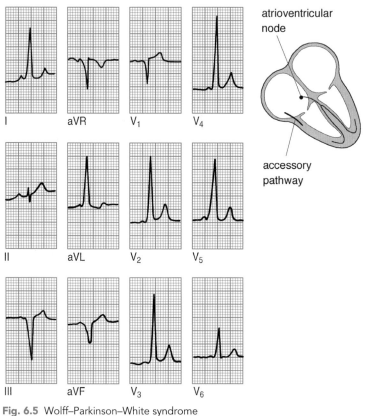

Fig. 6.5 Wolff–Parkinson–White syndrome

Key points: • short PR interval (0.08 s)
             • delta wave

WPW syndrome may be found incidentally and be asymptomatic – if so, no action is needed. Some patients develop palpitations due to an arrhythmia. The management of arrhythmias in WPW syndrome is discussed in detail on page 48. If a patient with WPW syndrome requires surgery of any kind, the anaesthetist must be informed of the ECG findings.

Lown–Ganong–Levine syndrome

Patients with LGL syndrome also have an accessory pathway (called the bundle of James). However, unlike the bundle of Kent in WPW syndrome, the bundle of James does not activate the ventricular muscle directly. Instead, it simply connects the atria to the bundle of His (Fig. 6.6).

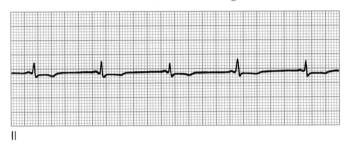

II

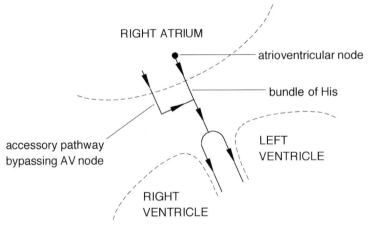

RIGHT ATRIUM

atrioventricular node

bundle of His

accessory pathway bypassing AV node

LEFT VENTRICLE

RIGHT VENTRICLE

Fig. 6.6 Lown–Ganong–Levine syndrome

Key points: ● short PR interval (0.08 s)
           ● no delta wave

Because the accessory bundle allows the wave of depolarization to bypass the slowly conducting AV node, patients with LGL syndrome have a short PR interval. However, as there is no abnormal ventricular activation, there is no delta wave. LGL syndrome carries the same risk of paroxysmal tachycardias as WPW syndrome.

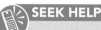

● Is the PR interval more than 0.2 s long?

Prolongation of the PR interval is a common finding and indicates that conduction through the AV node has been delayed. When this delay is constant for each cardiac cycle, and each P wave is followed by a QRS complex, it is referred to as **first-degree AV block**.

First-degree AV block is a common feature of vagally induced bradycardia, as an increase in vagal tone decreases AV nodal conduction. It may also be a feature of:

- ischaemic heart disease
- hypokalaemia
- acute rheumatic myocarditis
- Lyme disease
- drugs
    - digoxin
    - quinidine
    - beta blockers
    - rate-modifying calcium-channel blockers.

Figure 6.7 shows a rhythm strip from a patient with first-degree AV block.

Look for a cause by taking a thorough patient history and, in particular, asking about any drug treatment the patient is currently receiving.

First-degree AV block in itself is asymptomatic and, in general, does not progress to other sorts of heart block (these are described later). No specific treatment is necessary for first-degree AV block *in its own right*, but it should alert you to one of

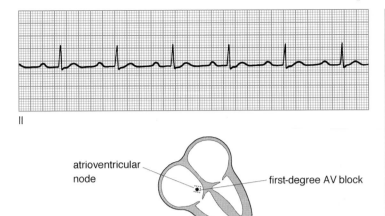

Fig. 6.7 First-degree AV block

Key point: • long PR interval (0.31 s)

the above diagnoses (which may require treatment). First-degree heart block is *not* an indication for a pacemaker.

● Does the PR interval vary or can it not be measured?

Normally, the PR interval is constant. In some conditions, however, the interval between P waves and QRS complexes changes, giving rise to a variable PR interval. Sometimes a P wave is not followed by a QRS complex at all and so the PR interval cannot be measured.

If either, or both, of these occur, they indicate one of several possible AV conduction problems. These are distinguished by the relationship between P waves and QRS complexes.

● If the PR interval gradually lengthens with each beat, until one P wave fails to produce a QRS complex, the patient has **Mobitz type I AV block**.

- If the PR interval is fixed and normal, but occasionally a P wave fails to produce a QRS complex, the patient has **Mobitz type II AV block**.
- If alternate P waves are not followed by QRS complexes, the patient has **2:1 AV block**.
- If there is no relationship between P waves and QRS complexes, the patient has **third-degree (complete) AV block**.

All these types of AV block are discussed below, with example ECGs.

Mobitz type I AV block

Mobitz type I AV block is one of the types of second-degree heart block and is also known as the Wenckebach phenomenon. Its characteristic features are:

- the PR interval shows progressive lengthening until one P wave fails to be conducted and fails to produce a QRS complex
- the PR interval resets to normal and the cycle repeats.

These features are demonstrated in the rhythm strip in Figure 6.8. Mobitz type I AV block is thought to result from abnormal conduction through the AV node itself and can result simply from periods of high vagal activity, so it sometimes occurs during sleep. It may also occur in generalized disease of the conducting tissues. It is regarded as a relatively benign form of AV block, and a permanent pacemaker is not required unless the frequency of 'dropped' ventricular beats causes a symptomatic bradycardia.

In acute myocardial infarction, however, pacing may be required, depending on the type of infarction. In **anterior** myocardial infarction, a prophylactic temporary pacemaker is recommended in case third-degree (complete) heart block develops. In **inferior** myocardial infarction, a pacemaker is only needed if symptoms or haemodynamic compromise result. Patients found to have

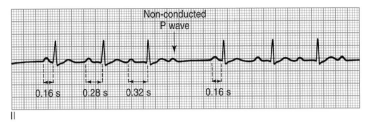

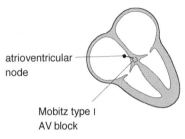

atrioventricular node

Mobitz type I
AV block

Fig. 6.8 Mobitz type I AV block

Key points:
- progressive lengthening of PR interval
- a P wave then fails to be conducted
- PR interval resets and cycle repeats

Mobitz type I AV block prior to surgery will usually require temporary pacing perioperatively – discuss this with the anaesthetist and a cardiologist.

 SEEK HELP

> Mobitz type I AV block may require pacing prior to surgery. Seek the advice of a cardiologist without delay.

Mobitz type II AV block

Mobitz type II AV block is another type of second-degree heart block and its characteristic features are:

- most P waves are followed by a QRS complex
- the PR interval is normal and constant
- occasionally, a P wave is not followed by a QRS complex.

These features are demonstrated in the rhythm strip in Figure 6.9.

Mobitz type II AV block is thought to result from abnormal conduction below the AV node, in the bundle of His, and is

121

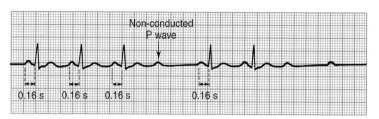

Non-conducted
P wave

0.16 s   0.16 s   0.16 s   0.16 s

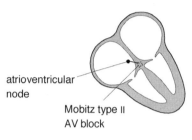

atrioventricular
node

Mobitz type II
AV block

Fig. 6.9 Mobitz type II AV block

Key point: • PR interval normal
and constant

considered more serious than Mobitz type I as it can progress
without warning to third-degree (complete) heart block.
Referral to a cardiologist is therefore recommended, as a pacemaker may be required.

The indications for pacing Mobitz type II AV block in the setting of an acute myocardial infarction, or perioperatively, are
the same as for Mobitz type I AV block.

 SEEK HELP

Mobitz type II AV block may require pacing. Seek the
advice of a cardiologist without delay.

2:1 AV block

2:1 AV block is a special form of second-degree heart block in
which alternate P waves are not followed by QRS complexes
(Fig. 6.10).

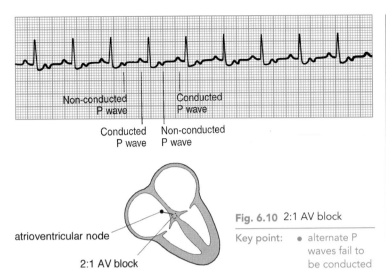

Non-conducted
P wave

Conducted
P wave

Conducted
P wave

Non-conducted
P wave

atrioventricular node

2:1 AV block

Fig. 6.10 2:1 AV block

Key point: • alternate P
waves fail to
be conducted

2:1 AV block cannot be categorized as Mobitz type I or type II because it is impossible to say whether the PR interval for the non-conducted P waves would have been the same as, or longer than, the conducted P waves.

Third-degree AV block

In third-degree AV block ('complete heart block'), there is complete interruption of conduction between atria and ventricles, so that the two are working independently. QRS complexes usually arise as the result of a ventricular escape rhythm (p. 59). An example is shown in Figure 6.11.

The characteristic features of complete heart block are:

- P wave rate is faster than ventricular QRS complexes
- P waves bear no relationship to the ventricular QRS complexes
- if block occurs in the AV node, QRS complexes are usually narrow due to a subsidiary pacemaker arising in the bundle of His

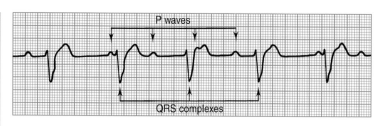

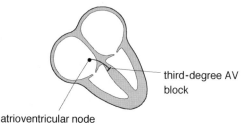

third-degree AV block

atrioventricular node

Fig. 6.11 Third-degree AV block

Key points:
- P wave (atrial) rate is 85/min
- QRS complex (ventricular) rate is 54/min
- broad QRS complexes
- no relationship between P waves and QRS complexes

- if block occurs below the AV node, QRS complexes are usually broad due to a subsidiary pacemaker arising in the left or right bundle branches.

It is important to remember that any atrial rhythm can coexist with third-degree heart block, and so the P waves may be abnormal or even absent. A combination of bradycardia (usually 15–40 beats/min) and broad QRS complexes should alert you to suspect third-degree heart block.

In acute **inferior** wall myocardial infarction, third-degree AV block requires pacing if the patient has symptoms or is haemodynamically compromised. In acute **anterior** wall myocardial infarction, the development of third-degree AV block usually indicates an extensive infarct (and thus a poor prognosis). Temporary pacing is indicated regardless of the patient's symptoms or haemodynamic state. Temporary pacing is also usually necessary perioperatively in patients about to undergo surgery who are found to have third-degree AV block.

In elderly people, third-degree AV block may cause heart failure, dizziness, falls or even loss of consciousness – permanent pacing is indicated under these circumstances.

Congenital varieties of third-degree AV block are uncommon and you should seek the advice of a cardiologist. In a young patient with a recent onset of third-degree AV block, always consider the possibility of Lyme disease. This is transmitted by the spirochaete *Borrelia burgdorferi* and, in the second stage of the illness, can lead to first-degree, second-degree or third-degree AV block. The AV block can resolve entirely in response to antibiotics, although the patient may require support with a temporary pacemaker during treatment.

SEEK HELP

Third-degree AV block usually requires pacing. Seek the advice of a cardiologist without delay.

● Atrioventricular dissociation

Atrioventricular dissociation is a term that is commonly used interchangeably with third-degree AV block; however, it does *not* mean the same thing. Atrioventricular dissociation occurs when the ventricular (QRS) rate is *higher* than the atrial (P wave) rate. The opposite is found in third-degree AV block. Atrioventricular dissociation usually occurs in the context of an escape rhythm (from the AV junction or ventricles) during sinus bradycardia, or an acceleration in a subsidiary focus in the AV junction or ventricles which then overtakes the sinoatrial node, which continues firing independently.

Summary

To assess the PR interval, ask the following questions:

1. Is the PR interval less than 0.12 s long?

If 'yes', consider:

- AV junctional rhythms
- WPW syndrome
- LGL syndrome.

2. Is the PR interval more than 0.2 s long?

If 'yes', consider:

- first-degree AV block
  - ischaemic heart disease
  - hypokalaemia
  - acute rheumatic myocarditis
  - Lyme disease
  - drugs (digoxin, quinidine, beta blockers, rate-modifying calcium-channel blockers).

3. Does the PR interval vary or can it not be measured?

If 'yes', consider:

- second-degree AV block
  - Mobitz type I (Wenckebach phenomenon)
  - Mobitz type II
  - 2:1 AV block
- third-degree AV block.

The Q wave

After measuring the PR interval, go on to examine the QRS complex in each lead. Begin by looking for Q waves. A Q wave is present whenever the first deflection of the QRS complex points downwards (Fig. 7.1).

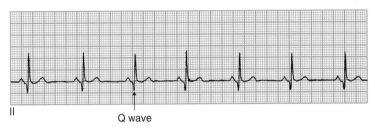

II

Q wave

Fig. 7.1 The Q wave

Key point: • Q wave is present when the first QRS deflection is downwards

As you examine the QRS complex in each lead for the Q wave, the question to ask is:

● Are there any 'pathological' Q waves?

In this chapter we will help you to answer this question and to interpret any abnormality you may find.

● Are there any 'pathological' Q waves?

If Q waves are present, begin by asking: Could these be normal?

Q waves are usually absent from *most* of the leads of a normal ECG. However, *small* Q waves (often referred to as q waves) are normal in leads that look at the heart from the left: I, II, aVL,

V_5 and V_6. They result from septal depolarization, which normally occurs from left to right, and hence are called 'septal' Q waves (Fig. 7.2).

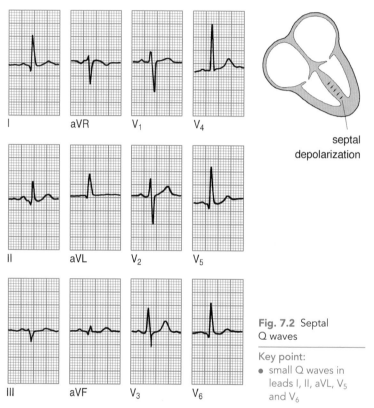

septal
depolarization

Fig. 7.2 Septal Q waves

Key point:
- small Q waves in leads I, II, aVL, V_5 and V_6

A small Q wave may be normal in lead III, and is often associated with an inverted T wave. Both may disappear on deep inspiration (Fig. 7.3). Q waves are also normal in lead aVR.

Q waves in other leads are likely to be abnormal or '*pathological*', particularly if they are:

- >2 small squares deep, or
- >25 per cent of the height of the following R wave in depth, and/or
- >1 small square wide.

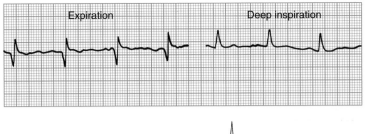

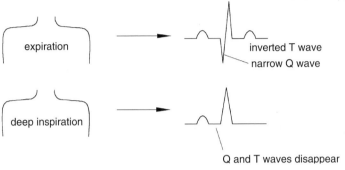

expiration → inverted T wave / narrow Q wave

deep inspiration → Q and T waves disappear

Fig. 7.3 Normal Q waves in lead III

Key points:
• narrow Q waves in lead III
• Q and T waves disappear on deep inspiration

If wide or deep Q waves (i.e. exceeding the above criteria) are present, consider:

• ST segment elevation myocardial infarction
• left ventricular hypertrophy
• Wolff–Parkinson–White syndrome
• bundle branch block.

Myocardial infarction, left ventricular hypertrophy and Wolff–Parkinson–White syndrome are discussed below. The bundle branch blocks are covered in detail in Chapter 8.

An abnormal Q wave (in lead III) is also a feature of:

• pulmonary embolism.

It is part of the 'classic' $S_I Q_{III} T_{III}$ pattern that is often quoted, although rarely seen. However, the Q_{III} rarely satisfies the 'pathological' Q wave criteria. The most frequent finding in pulmonary embolism is a tachycardia.

ST segment elevation myocardial infarction

Q waves start to appear within a few hours of the onset of ST segment elevation myocardial infarction and in 90 per cent of cases become permanent. The presence of Q waves alone therefore gives no clue about the timing of the infarction. As with the other ECG changes in myocardial infarction, the location of the infarct can be determined from an analysis of the ECG leads (see Table 9.2, p. 164).

Figure 7.4 shows an ECG recorded 5 days after an anterior myocardial infarction. Q waves have developed in leads V_1–V_4.

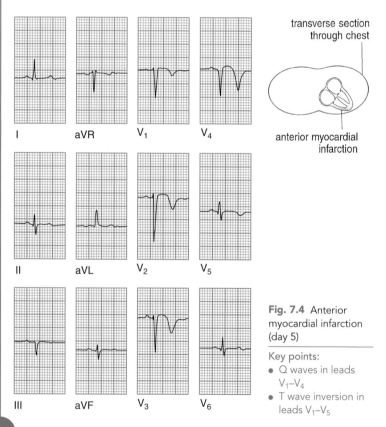

transverse section through chest

anterior myocardial infarction

Fig. 7.4 Anterior myocardial infarction (day 5)

Key points:
- Q waves in leads V_1–V_4
- T wave inversion in leads V_1–V_5

Figure 7.5 is from a patient who had an inferior myocardial infarction 2 years previously. Abnormal Q waves are seen in leads II, III and aVF.

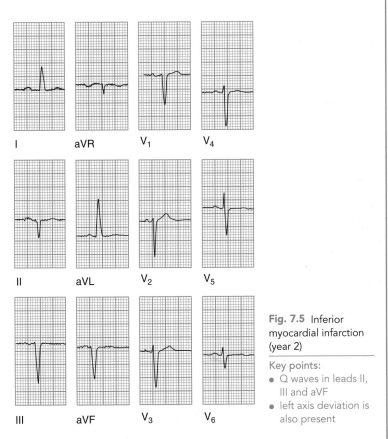

I   aVR   V$_1$ V$_4$

II   aVL   V$_2$ V$_5$

III   aVF   V$_3$ V$_6$

Fig. 7.5 Inferior myocardial infarction (year 2)

Key points:
- Q waves in leads II, III and aVF
- left axis deviation is also present

The diagnosis of acute myocardial infarction is usually apparent from the presenting symptoms (chest pain, nausea and sweating) and ECG changes that are present, and can be confirmed by serial cardiac marker measurements. The management of acute myocardial infarction is discussed in detail in Chapter 9.

ACT QUICKLY

Acute myocardial infarction is a medical emergency. Prompt diagnosis and treatment are essential.

● Why do Q waves appear in myocardial infarction?

Q waves develop in myocardial infarction following the necrosis (death) of an area of myocardium. The leads over the necrosed region can no longer record electrical activity in that area, and so they look 'through' it to record ventricular depolarization from 'within' the ventricular cavity rather than from outside.

Because each wave of depolarization flows from the inner surface of the heart to the outer, a lead recording the depolarization from a viewpoint 'within' the ventricle would 'see' the electrical activity flowing away from it; hence, the negative deflection on the ECG – the Q wave.

When Q waves are found 'incidentally' on an ECG recorded for other reasons, a thorough review of the patient's history is necessary. Ask about:

- previous documented myocardial infarctions
- previous symptoms suggestive of myocardial infarction
- symptoms of recent myocardial ischaemia.

However, bear in mind that approximately 20 per cent of myocardial infarctions are painless or 'silent'. If you remain uncertain about the importance of abnormal Q waves, and are suspicious about a previous myocardial infarction, there are many investigations that can help:

- exercise ECG (Chapter 16)
- echocardiography
- cardiac magnetic resonance imaging
- nuclear myocardial perfusion scan
- coronary angiography.

A cardiologist will be able to advise you on which of these tests, if any, are appropriate.

Left ventricular hypertrophy

At the start of this chapter, we said that small ('septal') Q waves can be a normal finding and result from depolarization of the interventricular septum. If the septum hypertrophies, its muscle mass (and hence the amount of electricity generated by depolarization) increases, and the Q waves become deeper.

Left ventricular hypertrophy often involves the septum, and so deep Q waves are often seen in leads looking at the left and inferior surfaces of the heart (Fig. 7.6).

Left ventricular hypertrophy is discussed more fully in Chapter 8.

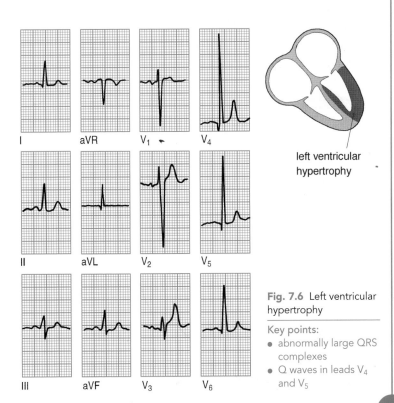

left ventricular
hypertrophy

Fig. 7.6 Left ventricular hypertrophy

Key points:
- abnormally large QRS complexes
- Q waves in leads V_4 and V_5

Wolff–Parkinson–White syndrome

The delta waves seen in Wolff–Parkinson–White syndrome, indicating ventricular pre-excitation, can be negative in some leads (depending on the location of the accessory pathway). As such, these negative delta waves can be mistaken for Q waves, particularly when they are seen inferiorly. This can lead to an incorrect diagnosis of myocardial infarction.

Wolff–Parkinson–White syndrome is discussed more fully in Chapter 6.

Summary

To assess the Q wave, ask the following question:

Are there any 'pathological' Q waves?

If 'yes', consider:

- ST segment elevation myocardial infarction
- left ventricular hypertrophy
- Wolff–Parkinson–White syndrome
- bundle branch block.

Also:

- pulmonary embolism (although rarely 'pathological').

8 The QRS complex

Normal QRS complexes have a different appearance in each of the 12 ECG leads (Fig. 8.1).

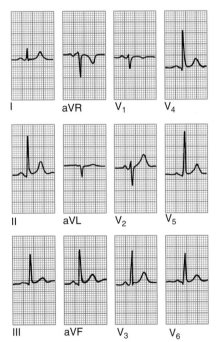

I aVR V₁ V₄

II aVL V₂ V₅

III aVF V₃ V₆

Fig. 8.1 Normal 12-lead ECG

Key point:
- appearance of QRS complex varies from lead to lead

When reviewing an ECG, look carefully at the size and shape of the QRS complexes in each lead and ask yourself the following four questions:

- Are any R or S waves too big?
- Are the QRS complexes too small?

- Are any QRS complexes too wide?
- Are any QRS complexes an abnormal shape?

In this chapter, we will help you to answer these questions and to interpret any abnormalities you may find.

● Are any R or S waves too big?

The height of the R wave and depth of the S wave vary from lead to lead in the normal ECG (as Fig. 8.1 shows). As a rule, in the normal ECG:

- the R wave *increases* in height from lead V_1 to V_5
- the R wave is *smaller* than the S wave in leads V_1 and V_2
- the R wave is *bigger* than the S wave in leads V_5 and V_6
- the tallest R wave does not exceed 25 mm in height
- the deepest S wave does not exceed 25 mm in depth.

Always look carefully at the R and S waves in each lead, and check whether they conform to these criteria. If not, first of all consider:

- ECG calibration (should be 1 mV = 10 mm).

If the calibration is correct, consider whether your patient has one of the following:

- left ventricular hypertrophy
- right ventricular hypertrophy
- posterior myocardial infarction
- Wolff–Parkinson–White syndrome
- dextrocardia.

Each of these conditions is discussed below.

If the QRS complex is also abnormally wide, think of:

- bundle branch block (discussed later in this chapter).

Left ventricular hypertrophy

Hypertrophy of the left ventricle causes tall R waves in the leads that 'look at' the left ventricle – I, aVL, V_5 and V_6 – and the reciprocal ('mirror image') change of deep S waves in leads that 'look at' the right ventricle – V_1 and V_2.

There are many criteria for the ECG diagnosis of left ventricular hypertrophy, with varying sensitivity and specificity. Generally, the diagnostic criteria are quite specific (if the criteria are present, the likelihood of the patient having left ventricular hypertrophy is >90 per cent), but not sensitive (the criteria will fail to detect 40–80 per cent of patients with left ventricular hypertrophy). The diagnostic criteria include:

- In the limb leads:
  - R wave greater than 11 mm in lead aVL
  - R wave greater than 20 mm in lead aVF
  - S wave greater than 14 mm in lead aVR
  - sum of R wave in lead I and S wave in lead III greater than 25 mm.
- In the chest leads:
  - R wave of 25 mm or more in the left chest leads
  - S wave of 25 mm or more in the right chest leads
  - sum of S wave in lead V_1 and R wave in lead V_5 or V_6 greater than 35 mm (Sokolow–Lyon criterion)
  - sum of tallest R wave and deepest S wave in the chest leads greater than 45 mm.

The **Cornell criteria** involve measuring the S wave in lead V_3 and the R wave in lead aVL. Left ventricular hypertrophy is indicated by a sum of >28 mm in men and >20 mm in women.

The **Romhilt–Estes scoring system** allocates points for the presence of certain criteria. A score of 5 indicates left ventricular hypertrophy and a score of 4 indicates probable left ventricular hypertrophy. Points are allocated as follows:

- 3 points – for (a) R or S wave in limb leads of 20 mm or more, (b) S wave in right chest leads of 25 mm or more, or (c) R wave in left chest leads of 25 mm or more

- 3 points – for ST segment and T wave changes ('typical strain') in a patient not taking digitalis (1 point with digitalis)
- 3 points – for P-terminal force in V_1 greater than 1 mm deep with a duration greater than 0.04 s
- 2 points – for left axis deviation (beyond –15°)
- 1 point – QRS complex duration greater than >0.09 s
- 1 point – intrinsicoid deflection (the interval from the start of the QRS complex to the peak of the R wave) in V_5 or V_6 greater than 0.05 s.

Figure 8.2 shows the ECG of a patient with left ventricular hypertrophy.

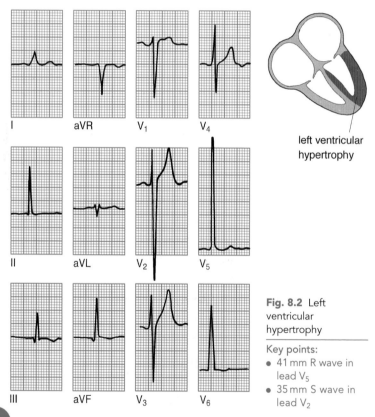

left ventricular hypertrophy

Fig. 8.2 Left ventricular hypertrophy

Key points:
- 41 mm R wave in lead V_5
- 35 mm S wave in lead V_2

If there is no evidence of left ventricular hypertrophy on the ECG, look for evidence of 'strain':

- ST segment depression
- T wave inversion.

(See Figure 9.16 for an example of left ventricular hypertrophy with 'strain'.)

Echocardiography is diagnostic for left ventricular hypertrophy. The treatment is usually that of the cause (Table 8.1).

Table 8.1 Causes of left ventricular hypertrophy

- Hypertension
- Aortic stenosis
- Coarctation of the aorta
- Hypertrophic cardiomyopathy

Right ventricular hypertrophy

Right ventricular hypertrophy causes a 'dominant' R wave (i.e. bigger than the S wave) in the leads that 'look at' the right ventricle, particularly V_1. Right ventricular hypertrophy is also associated with:

- right axis deviation (see Chapter 4)
- deep S waves in leads V_5 and V_6
- right bundle branch block (RBBB).

and, if 'strain' is present:

- ST segment depression
- T wave inversion.

Figure 8.3 shows the ECG of a patient with right ventricular hypertrophy and 'strain'.

If you suspect right ventricular hypertrophy, look for an underlying cause (Table 8.2). The treatment of right ventricular hypertrophy is that of the underlying cause.

Posterior myocardial infarction

Posterior myocardial infarction is one of the few causes of a 'dominant' R wave in lead V_1 (Table 8.3).

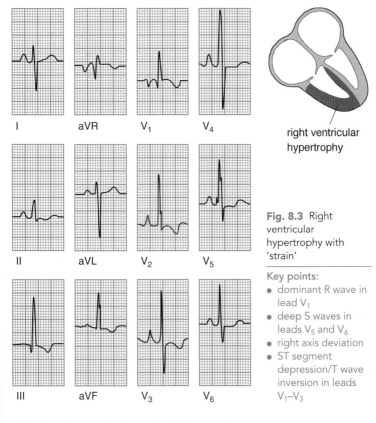

I aVR V₁ V₄

II aVL V₂ V₅

III aVF V₃ V₆

right ventricular
hypertrophy

Fig. 8.3 Right
ventricular
hypertrophy with
'strain'

Key points:
- dominant R wave in
  lead V₁
- deep S waves in
  leads V₅ and V₆
- right axis deviation
- ST segment
  depression/T wave
  inversion in leads
  V₁–V₃

Table 8.2 Causes of right ventricular hypertrophy

- Pulmonary hypertension
- Pulmonary stenosis

Table 8.3 Causes of a 'dominant' R wave in lead V₁

- Right ventricular hypertrophy
- Posterior myocardial infarction
- Wolff–Parkinson–White syndrome (left-sided accessory pathway)

Infarction of the posterior wall of the left ventricle leads to reciprocal changes when viewed from the perspective of the anterior chest leads. Thus, the usual appearances of pathological

Q waves, ST segment elevation and inverted T waves will appear as *R waves*, ST segment *depression* and *upright, tall* T waves when viewed from leads V_1–V_3 (Fig. 8.4).

The management of acute myocardial infarction is discussed in detail in Chapter 9.

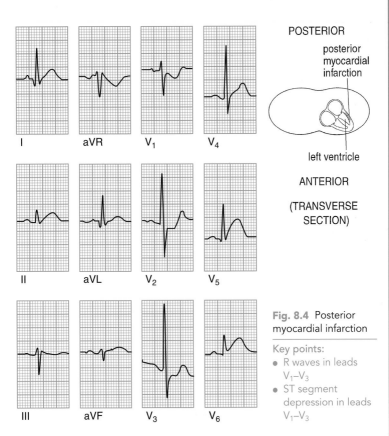

I aVR V_1 V_4

II aVL V_2 V_5

III aVF V_3 V_6

POSTERIOR

posterior myocardial infarction

left ventricle

ANTERIOR

(TRANSVERSE SECTION)

Fig. 8.4 Posterior myocardial infarction

Key points:
- R waves in leads V_1–V_3
- ST segment depression in leads V_1–V_3

ACT QUICKLY

Acute myocardial infarction is a medical emergency. Prompt diagnosis and treatment are essential.

Wolff–Parkinson–White syndrome

If you see a dominant R wave in leads V_1–V_3 in the presence of a short PR interval, think of Wolff–Parkinson–White syndrome (p. 114). Patients with Wolff–Parkinson–White syndrome have an accessory pathway (the bundle of Kent) that bypasses the atrioventricular node and bundle of His to connect the atria directly to the ventricles.

The position of the accessory pathway can be accurately localized only with electrophysiological studies. Generally, however, a dominant R wave in leads V_1–V_3 indicates a left-sided accessory pathway, whereas a dominant S wave in leads V_1–V_3 indicates a right-sided accessory pathway.

The management of Wolff–Parkinson–White syndrome is discussed in Chapter 6.

Dextrocardia

In dextrocardia, the heart lies on the right side of the chest instead of the left. The ECG does not show the normal progressive increase in R wave height across the chest leads; instead, the QRS complexes decrease in height across them (Fig. 8.5). In addition, the P wave is inverted in lead I and there is right axis deviation. **Right-sided chest leads** will show the pattern normally seen on the left.

If you suspect dextrocardia, check the location of the patient's apex beat. A chest radiograph is diagnostic. No specific treatment is required for dextrocardia, but ensure the condition is highlighted in the patient's notes and check for any associated syndromes (e.g. Kartagener's syndrome – dextrocardia, bronchiectasis and sinusitis).

● Are the QRS complexes too small?

Small QRS complexes indicate that relatively little of the voltage generated by ventricular depolarization is reaching the

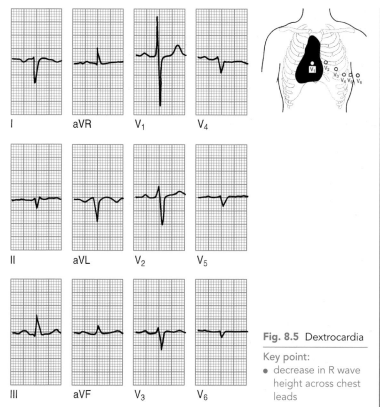

I	aVR	V₁	V₄
II	aVL	V₂	V₅
III	aVF	V₃	V₆

Fig. 8.5 Dextrocardia

Key point:
● decrease in R wave height across chest leads

ECG electrodes. Although criteria exist for the normal upper limit of QRS complex size, there are no similar guidelines for the lower limit of QRS size.

Small QRS complexes may simply reflect a variant of normal. However, always check for:

● ECG calibration (should be 1 mV = 10 mm).

Also check whether the patient has:

● obesity
● emphysema.

Both of these conditions increase the distance between the heart and the chest electrodes.

However, if the QRS complexes appear small, and particularly if they have changed in relation to earlier ECG recordings, always consider the possibility of:

● pericardial effusion.

This is discussed below.

Pericardial effusion

Pericardial effusion reduces the voltage of the QRS complexes (Fig. 8.6).

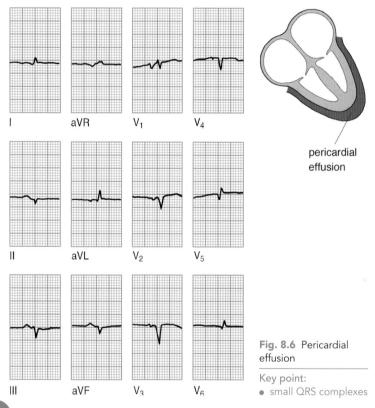

pericardial
effusion

Fig. 8.6 Pericardial effusion

Key point:
● small QRS complexes

Pericardial effusion can also cause electrical alternans, in which the height of the R waves and/or T waves alternates from beat to beat (Fig. 8.7).

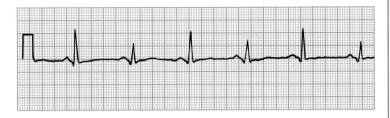

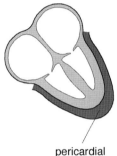

Fig. 8.7 Electrical alternans in pericardial effusion

pericardial effusion

Key point: ● variation in beat-to-beat R wave height

Pericardial effusion may be asymptomatic when small. Larger effusions cause breathlessness and, ultimately, cardiac tamponade. The presence of Beck's triad indicates major cardiac compromise:

● low blood pressure
● elevated jugular venous pressure
● impalpable apex beat.

In addition, the heart sounds are soft and there may be pulsus paradoxus (a marked fall in blood pressure on inspiration). The combination of small QRS complexes, electrical alternans and a tachycardia is a highly specific, but insensitive, indicator of a pericardial tamponade.

In a patient with a pericardial effusion, the chest radiograph may show a large globular heart but with no distension of the pulmonary veins. The echocardiogram is diagnostic.

Obtain the advice of a cardiologist immediately, particularly if the effusion is causing haemodynamic impairment. Urgent pericardial aspiration is required if the signs of tamponade are present, but should only be undertaken by, or under the guidance of, someone experienced in the procedure.

ACT QUICKLY

Cardiac tamponade is a medical emergency. Prompt diagnosis and treatment are essential.

● Are any QRS complexes too wide?

The QRS complex corresponds to depolarization of the ventricles, and this normally takes no longer than 0.12 s from start to finish. Thus, the width of a normal QRS complex is no greater than 3 small squares on the ECG.

Widening of the QRS complex is seen if conduction through the ventricles is slower than normal, and this usually means that depolarization has taken an abnormal route through the ventricles, as happens in:

- bundle branch block
- ventricular rhythms.

These conditions are discussed below.

Widening of the QRS complex can also result from the abnormal mechanism of depolarization that occurs with:

- hyperkalaemia.

Hyperkalaemia is discussed in detail on page 187.

Bundle branch block

After leaving the bundle of His, the conduction fibres divide into two pathways as they pass through the interventricular septum – the left and right bundle branches, which supply the left and right ventricles, respectively.

A block of either of the bundle branches delays the electrical activation of its ventricle, which must instead be depolarized *indirectly* via the other bundle branch. This prolongs the process of ventricular depolarization, and so the QRS complex is wider than 3 small squares. In addition, the shape of the QRS complex is distorted because of the abnormal pathway of depolarization.

In **left bundle branch block** (LBBB), the interventricular septum has to depolarize from right to left, a reversal of the normal pattern. This causes a small Q wave in lead V_1 and a small R wave in lead V_6 (Fig. 8.8). The right ventricle is depolarized normally via the right bundle branch, causing an R wave in lead V_1 and an S wave in lead V_6 (Fig. 8.9). Then, the left ventricle is depolarized by the right, causing an S wave in lead V_1 and another R wave (called R′) in lead V_6 (Fig. 8.10).

Thus, the ECG of a patient with LBBB appears as in Figure 8.11.

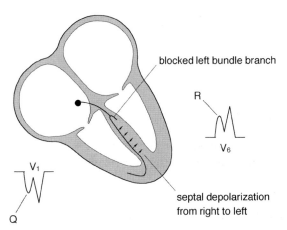

blocked left bundle branch

R

V_6

septal depolarization from right to left

V_1

Q

Fig. 8.8 Left bundle branch block (1)

Key points:
- septal depolarization occurs from right to left
- small Q wave in lead V_1
- small R wave in lead V_6

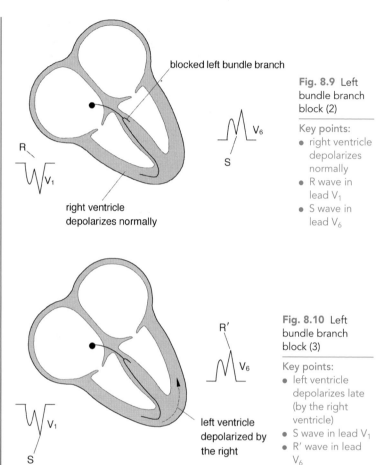

Fig. 8.9 Left bundle branch block (2)

Key points:
- right ventricle depolarizes normally
- R wave in lead V_1
- S wave in lead V_6

Fig. 8.10 Left bundle branch block (3)

Key points:
- left ventricle depolarizes late (by the right ventricle)
- S wave in lead V_1
- R′ wave in lead V_6

In **right bundle branch block**, the interventricular septum depolarizes normally, from left to right, causing a tiny R wave in lead V_1 and a small 'septal' Q wave in lead V_6 (Fig. 8.12). The left ventricle is depolarized normally via the left bundle branch, causing an S wave in lead V_1 and an R wave in lead V_6 (Fig. 8.13).

Then, the right ventricle is depolarized by the left, causing another R wave (called R′) in lead V_1 and an S wave in lead V_6 (Fig. 8.14).

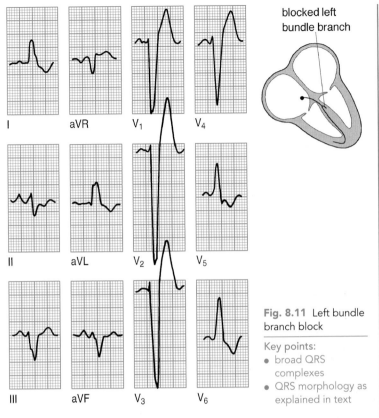

blocked left
bundle branch

Fig. 8.11 Left bundle
branch block

Key points:
- broad QRS
  complexes
- QRS morphology as
  explained in text

Thus, the ECG of a patient with RBBB appears as in Figure 8.15.

An aide-mémoire

Remembering the name 'William Morrow' should help you recall that:

- In LBBB, the QRS looks like a 'W' in lead V_1 and an 'M' in lead V_6 (**William**).
- In RBBB, the QRS looks like an 'M' in lead V_1 and a 'W' in lead V_6 (**Morrow**).

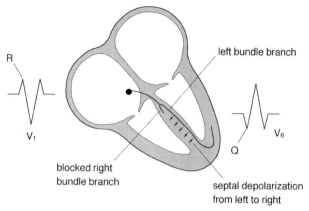

Fig. 8.12 Right bundle branch block (1)

Key points:
- septal depolarization occurs from left to right
- small R wave in lead V_1
- small 'septal' Q wave in lead V_6

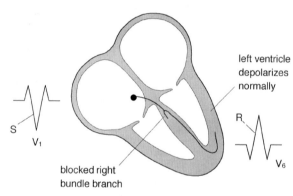

Fig. 8.13 Right bundle branch block (2)

Key points:
- left ventricle depolarizes normally
- S wave in lead V_1
- R wave in lead V_6

The presence of LBBB is almost invariably an indication of underlying pathology (Table 8.4), and the patient should be assessed accordingly. LBBB can be the presenting ECG feature of acute myocardial infarction, and is an indication for

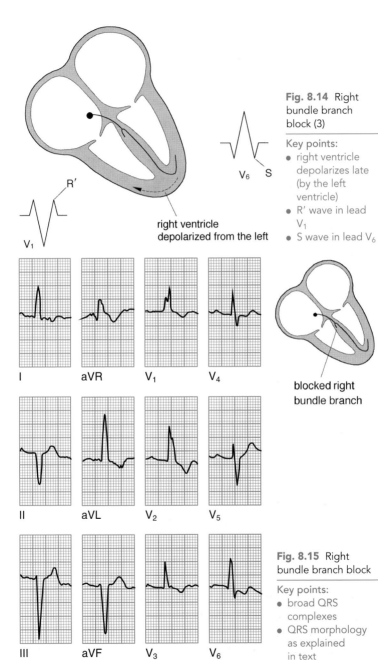

Fig. 8.14 Right bundle branch block (3)

Key points:
- right ventricle depolarizes late (by the left ventricle)
- R' wave in lead V₁
- S wave in lead V₆

right ventricle depolarized from the left

blocked right bundle branch

Fig. 8.15 Right bundle branch block

Key points:
- broad QRS complexes
- QRS morphology as explained in text

Table 8.4 Causes of left bundle branch block

- Ischaemic heart disease
- Cardiomyopathy
- Left ventricular hypertrophy
  - Hypertension
  - Aortic stenosis
- Fibrosis of the conduction system

thrombolysis. The presence of LBBB renders interpretation of the ECG beyond the QRS complex impossible.

In contrast with LBBB, RBBB is a relatively common finding in otherwise normal hearts. However, it too can result from underlying disease (Table 8.5) and should be investigated according to the clinical presentation.

Table 8.5 Causes of right bundle branch block

- Ischaemic heart disease
- Cardiomyopathy
- Atrial septal defect
- Ebstein's anomaly
- Pulmonary embolism (usually massive)

Bundle branch block (particularly RBBB) can also occur at fast heart rates. This is not uncommonly seen during supraventricular tachycardia (SVT), and the resultant broad complexes can lead to an incorrect diagnosis of ventricular tachycardia (VT) by the unwary. For help in distinguishing between VT and SVT, see page 74.

Both LBBB and RBBB are asymptomatic in themselves, and do not require treatment in their own right. Even so, they should prompt you to look for an underlying cause that is appropriate to the patient's presentation.

Ventricular rhythms

When depolarization is initiated from within the ventricular muscle itself, the wave of electrical activity has to spread from myocyte to myocyte rather than using the more rapid Purkinje network. This prolongs the process of ventricular depolarization and thus widens the QRS complex (Fig. 8.16).

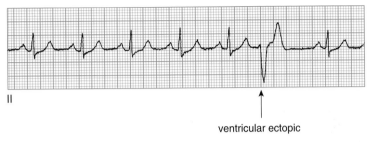

ventricular ectopic

Fig. 8.16 Ventricular ectopic

Key points:
- broad QRS complex
- complex occurs earlier than expected

For more information about ventricular rhythms, and help with their identification, see Chapter 3.

● Are any QRS complexes an abnormal shape?

Most of the causes of an abnormally shaped QRS complex have been discussed earlier in this chapter. However, occasionally you will encounter QRS complexes that just appear unusual, without fitting any of the specific criteria mentioned above.

You may see complexes which appear 'slurred', or have an abnormal 'notch', without necessarily being abnormally tall, small or wide. If this is the case, consider the following possible causes:

- incomplete bundle branch block
- fascicular block
- Wolff–Parkinson–White syndrome.

Further information on each of these can be found below.

Incomplete bundle branch block

Bundle branch block is discussed earlier in this chapter. Sometimes, however, conduction down a bundle branch can be *delayed* without being blocked entirely. When this happens, the QRS complex develops an abnormal shape but the complex remains less than 3 small squares wide. This is called incomplete (or partial) bundle branch block, and can affect either the left or the right bundle branches (Figs. 8.17 and 8.18).

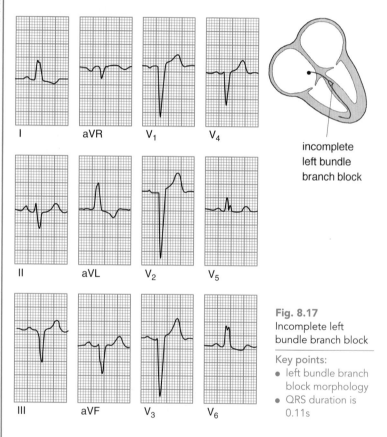

incomplete
left bundle
branch block

Fig. 8.17
Incomplete left
bundle branch block

Key points:
- left bundle branch block morphology
- QRS duration is 0.11s

The causes of incomplete bundle branch block are the same as those of complete bundle branch block, discussed earlier in this chapter.

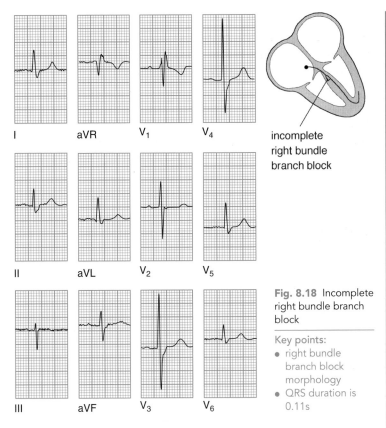

I   aVR   V₁   V₄

incomplete
right bundle
branch block

II   aVL   V₂   V₅

Fig. 8.18 Incomplete
right bundle branch
block

Key points:
- right bundle
  branch block
  morphology
- QRS duration is
  0.11s

III   aVF   V₃   V₆

Fascicular block

Block of one of the two fascicles of the left bundle causes either left or right axis deviation (Chapter 4). The consequent delay to conduction may also lead to slurring or notching of the QRS complex.

How to identify which fascicle is affected, and manage the patient subsequently, is discussed in Chapter 4.

Wolff–Parkinson–White syndrome

Patients with Wolff–Parkinson–White syndrome characteristically exhibit a delta wave that slurs the upstroke of the QRS complex (see Fig. 6.4, p. 115). This diagnosis should be suspected if, in addition, the PR interval is abnormally short. For more information on the diagnosis and management of Wolff–Parkinson–White syndrome, see page 114.

Summary

To assess the QRS complex, ask the following questions:

1. Are any R or S waves too big?

If 'yes', consider:

- incorrect ECG calibration
- left ventricular hypertrophy
- right ventricular hypertrophy
- posterior myocardial infarction
- Wolff–Parkinson–White syndrome (left-sided accessory pathway)
- dextrocardia.

Also:

- bundle branch block.

2. Are the QRS complexes too small?

If 'yes', consider:

- incorrect ECG calibration
- obesity
- emphysema
- pericardial effusion.

3. Are any QRS complexes too wide?

If 'yes', consider:

- bundle branch block
- ventricular rhythms.

Also:

- hyperkalaemia.

4. Are any QRS complexes an abnormal shape?

If 'yes', consider:

- incomplete bundle branch block
- fascicular block
- Wolff–Parkinson–White syndrome.

The ST segment 9

The ST segment lies between the end of the S wave and the start of the T wave. Normally, the ST segment is isoelectric, meaning that it lies at the same level as the ECG's baseline, the horizontal line between the end of the T wave and the start of the P wave (Fig. 9.1).

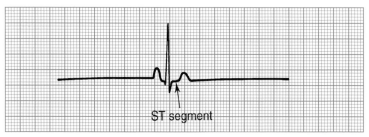

ST segment

Fig. 9.1 The ST segment

Key point: • ST segment is normally isoelectric

ST segments can be abnormal in one of three ways, so the questions you need to ask about the ST segments when you review them are:

- Are the ST segments elevated?
- Are the ST segments depressed?
- Are J waves present?

In this chapter, we will help you to answer these questions, and guide you about what to do next if you find an abnormality.

● Are the ST segments elevated?

Look carefully at the ST segment in each lead to see if it is isoelectric. If it is raised above this level, the ST segment is elevated.

ST segment elevation should never be ignored, as it often indicates a serious problem that warrants urgent attention. If you see ST elevation in any lead, consider the following possible diagnoses:

● ST segment elevation acute coronary syndrome
● left ventricular aneurysm
● Prinzmetal's (vasospastic) angina
● pericarditis
● high take-off
● left bundle branch block
● Brugada syndrome.

Therefore, ST segment elevation can represent anything from a potentially life-threatening condition to a normal variant, making it particularly important to identify the cause. To help you in this task, we describe each of these conditions (together with example ECGs) below.

ST segment elevation acute coronary syndrome

Patients presenting with acute coronary ischaemic syndromes have traditionally been divided into those with myocardial infarction and those with unstable angina. The problem with this is that a diagnosis of myocardial infarction requires the detection of myocardial damage, usually shown by a rise in circulating levels of markers of myocyte necrosis (e.g. troponin T or I, creatine kinase), and this takes time. It can take 12 hours for levels of cardiac markers to rise markedly. However, important therapeutic decisions need to be taken early on. A more helpful way of categorizing acute coronary syndromes is on the basis of the presenting ECG changes, and in particular whether ST segment elevation is present or not. In this way, patients presenting with an acute coronary syndrome can be divided into two groups:

- ST segment elevation acute coronary syndrome (STEACS)
- non-ST segment elevation acute coronary syndrome (NSTEACS).

Patients with NSTEACS may present with ST segment depression, T wave inversion or no acute ECG changes at all.

Later on during the patient's admission, when the levels of blood cardiac markers become known, the diagnosis can be refined. The subgroup of patients with raised cardiac markers can be recategorized into:

- ST segment elevation myocardial infarction (STEMI)
- non-ST segment elevation myocardial infarction (NSTEMI).

Those whose cardiac markers are not raised can continue to be categorized as STEACS and NSTEACS, or more generally as either 'acute coronary syndrome' or 'unstable angina'.

This section is chiefly concerned with STEACS. More information about NSTEACS can be found in Chapter 10.

In STEACS, the ECG changes gradually 'evolve' in the sequence shown in Figure 9.2. The earliest change is ST segment elevation accompanied, or even preceded, by tall 'hyperacute' T waves. Over the next few hours or days, Q waves appear, the ST segments return to normal and the T waves become inverted. It is usual for some permanent abnormality of the ECG to persist following STEACS – usually 'pathological' Q waves, although the T waves may remain inverted permanently too.

Do not forget that acute myocardial infarction can also present with the new onset of left bundle branch block on the ECG (Chapter 8). Also, a normal ECG does not exclude an acute myocardial infarction.

ST segment elevation acute coronary syndrome requires urgent treatment and you must not lose any time in trying to make the diagnosis. An urgent ECG is therefore needed in patients

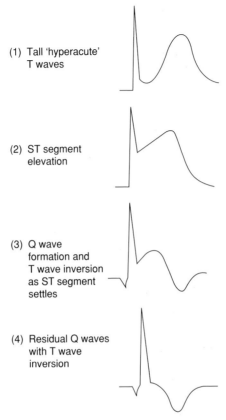

(1) Tall 'hyperacute' T waves

(2) ST segment elevation

(3) Q wave formation and T wave inversion as ST segment settles

(4) Residual Q waves with T wave inversion

Fig. 9.2 Evolution of a Q wave myocardial infarction

presenting with chest pain suggestive of myocardial ischaemia. The key symptoms of an acute coronary syndrome are:

- tight, central chest pain
- nausea and vomiting
- sweating.

The pain is more severe, and longer lasting, than that of angina. Always ask about a history of previous angina or myocardial infarction and assess cardiac risk factors (Table 9.1) and any possible contraindications to aspirin or thrombolysis. A thorough clinical examination is mandatory.

Table 9.1 Risk factors for coronary artery disease

Modifiable:
- Cigarette smoking
- Hypertension
- Diabetes mellitus
- Dyslipidaemia
- Overweight and obesity
- Physical inactivity

Non-modifiable:
- Age
- Male sex
- Family history

- **Aortic dissection**
  Beware of missing a diagnosis of aortic dissection. This too can cause ST segment elevation (if the dissection involves the coronary arteries) and chest pain, but patients may also complain of a 'tearing' back pain with different blood pressure in each arm, and a chest radiograph will show mediastinal widening.

Cardiac markers commonly measured to detect myocardial infarction are:

- troponins I and T
- creatine kinase (CK) or its isoenzyme CK-MB (which is more cardiac specific).

Other cardiac markers which are elevated in myocardial infarction (but which are less commonly used diagnostically nowadays) include:

- aspartate transaminase (AST)
- lactate dehydrogenase (LDH).

Troponins are relatively sensitive and specific markers of myocyte necrosis. The isoenzyme CK-MB is more cardiac specific than CK, AST or LDH.

Cardiac markers peak at different times after the onset of the infarction (Fig. 9.3). You can see from Figure 9.3 that marked changes in the cardiac enzymes may not be apparent until several hours after the onset of an infarction. Cardiac markers therefore have little role in the initial diagnosis of a myocardial infarction, and it is not at all unusual for levels to be normal on admission. The diagnosis of STEACS is therefore based on the presenting history and ECG changes; confirmation of whether myocardial infarction has occurred takes place later, when the cardiac marker results become available.

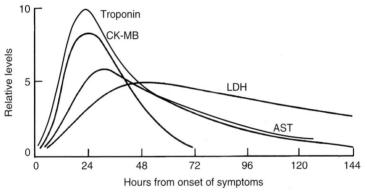

Fig. 9.3 Time course of enzyme levels after myocardial infarction

Key points:
- Troponins peak after 18–24 h
- CK-MB peaks after 24 h
- AST peaks after 30 h
- LDH peaks after 48 h

Having diagnosed STEACS, waste no time in admitting the patient to a coronary care unit or other monitored area for treatment as indicated. This is discussed later in this section.

The ECG also allows you to identify the area of myocardium affected by STEACS, as the leads 'looking at' that area will be the ones in which abnormalities are seen (Table 9.2). Examples of ST segment elevation in different myocardial territories are shown in Figures 9.4–9.6.

Table 9.2 Localization of ST segment elevation acute coronary syndrome

Leads containing ST segment elevation	Location of event
V_1–V_4	Anterior
I, aVL, V_5–V_6	Lateral
I, aVL, V_1–V_6	Anterolateral
V_1–V_3	Anteroseptal
II, III, aVF	Inferior
I, aVL, V_5–V_6, II, III, aVF	Inferolateral

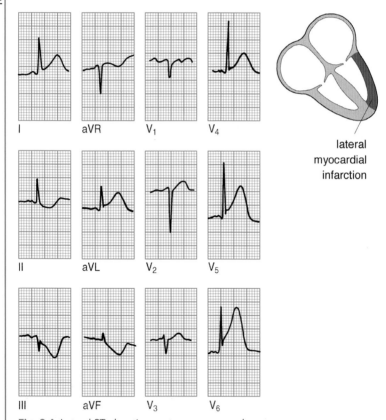

lateral myocardial infarction

Fig. 9.4 Lateral ST elevation acute coronary syndrome

Key points:
- ST segment elevation in leads I, aVL, and V_5–V_6
- 'hyperacute' T waves in leads V_5 and V_6

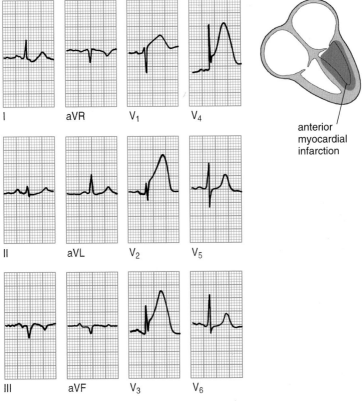

anterior
myocardial
infarction

Fig. 9.5 Anterior ST elevation acute coronary syndrome

Key point: • ST segment elevation in leads V_1–V_4

If you diagnose an inferior STEACS, you must go on to ask the question:

• Is the right ventricle involved?

To make the diagnosis, you must take another ECG, but this time use right-sided chest leads (Fig. 9.7). Look for ST segment elevation in lead V_4R (Fig. 9.8). If present, there is a high likelihood of right ventricular involvement.

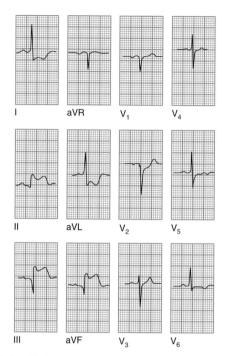

Fig. 9.6 Inferior ST elevation acute coronary syndrome

Key points:
- ST segment elevation in leads II, III and aVF
- reciprocal ST segment depression in leads I and aVL

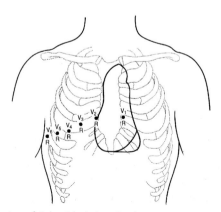

Fig. 9.7 Positioning of right-sided chest leads

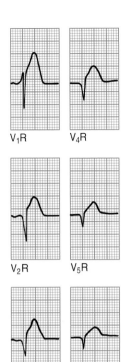

V₁R V₄R

V₂R V₅R

V₃R V₆R

Fig. 9.8 Right ventricular involvement

Key points:
- only right-sided chest leads are shown
- ST segment elevation in all leads (including V₄R)

Patients with STEACS require:

- pain relief (an opioid intravenously and an anti-emetic)
- oxygen
- aspirin, 300 mg orally
- clopidogrel, 300 mg orally.

Urgent myocardial reperfusion is the main priority in STEACS. This can be achieved by primary percutaneous coronary intervention (PCI) or, if facilities for coronary angiography and primary PCI are unavailable, by intravenous administration of a thrombolytic agent. Thrombolysis is indicated

● Why is right ventricular infarction important?

Patients with right ventricular infarction may develop the signs of right-sided heart failure (elevated jugular venous pressure and peripheral oedema). The left ventricle may be functioning normally, so the lungs are clear. If these patients develop hypotension, it is usually because their left-sided filling pressure is too low (as the supply of blood from the damaged right ventricle is inadequate). Vasodi-lator drugs must be avoided. Intravenous fluids may be needed to maintain right ventricular output, thus ensuring sufficient blood is supplied to the left ventricle.

It may seem paradoxical to give intravenous fluids to patients who already appear to be in right heart failure, unless the reasons for doing so are understood. If haemodynamically compromised, these patients need fluid balance monitoring using a Swan–Ganz catheter, which measures right-sided and, indirectly, left-sided filling pressure. The risk of severe complications is high in these patients.

(unless contraindicated) in patients whose history suggests a myocardial infarction within the past 12 h and whose ECG shows:

- ST segment elevation consistent with infarction, or
- new left bundle branch block.

Following STEACS, patients should continue with:

- aspirin, 75 mg daily
- clopidogrel, 75 mg daily (short term)
- a beta blocker (e.g. timolol, 5 mg twice daily)
- an angiotensin-converting enzyme inhibitor
- a statin.

Left ventricular aneurysm

The development of a left ventricular aneurysm is a late complication of myocardial infarction, seen (to varying degrees) in about 10 per cent of survivors. The presence of an aneurysm can lead to persistent ST segment elevation in those chest leads that 'look at' the affected region (Fig. 9.9).

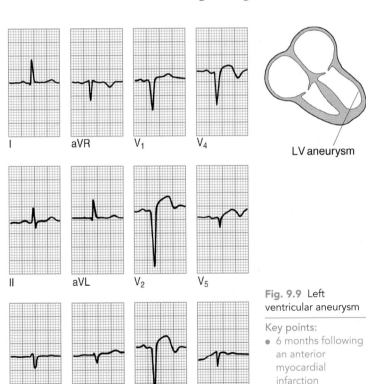

LV aneurysm

Fig. 9.9 Left ventricular aneurysm

Key points:
- 6 months following an anterior myocardial infarction
- persistent ST segment elevation in leads V_1–V_5

Ask the patient about a history of previous myocardial infarction and assess the patient for symptoms and signs related to the aneurysm itself. Aneurysms, being non-contractile, can lead to left ventricular dysfunction and thrombus formation. They can also be a focus for arrhythmia generation. Presenting symptoms can result from:

- heart failure
- embolic events
- arrhythmias.

The clinical signs of a left ventricular aneurysm are a 'double impulse' on precordial palpation and a fourth heart sound on auscultation. A chest radiograph may reveal a bulge on the cardiac outline. The investigation of choice is echocardiography, which will reveal the site of the aneurysm and the presence of mural thrombus, as well as allowing assessment of overall left ventricular function.

Patients with left ventricular aneurysms may benefit from treatment for heart failure and use of anticoagulation and anti-arrhythmic drugs. Consideration may also be given to surgical removal of the aneurysm (aneurysmectomy) or even cardiac transplantation where appropriate. Specialist referral is therefore recommended.

 SEEK HELP

A left ventricular aneurysm warrants specialist assessment. Obtain the advice of a cardiologist without delay.

Prinzmetal's (vasospastic) angina

Prinzmetal's angina refers to reversible myocardial ischaemia that results from coronary artery spasm. Although it can occur with normal coronary arteries, in over 90 per cent of cases the spasm is superimposed on some degree of atherosclerosis. Although any artery can be affected, spasm most commonly occurs in the right coronary artery. During an episode of vasospasm, the patient develops ST segment elevation in the affected territory (Fig. 9.10).

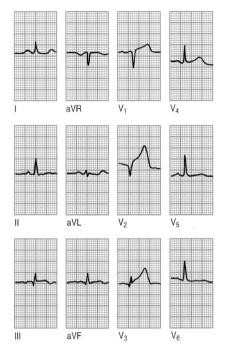

I	aVR	V₁	V₄
II	aVL	V₂	V₅
III	aVF	V₃	V₆

Fig. 9.10 Prinzmetal's (vasospastic) angina

Key points:
- anterior ST segment elevation during episode of chest pain

Although the combination of chest pain and ST segment elevation often suggests myocardial infarction, vasospastic angina is distinguished by the transient nature of the ST segment elevation. Unlike myocardial infarction, the ECG changes of vasospastic angina resolve entirely when the episode of chest pain settles. Ask the patient about prior episodes of chest pain, which typically occur at rest and particularly overnight in vasospastic angina. Patients may also have a history of other vasospastic disorders, such as Raynaud's phenomenon.

The ST segment elevation of vasospastic angina may be accompanied by tall 'hyperacute' T waves or, sometimes, T wave inversion. Transient intraventricular conduction defects, such as a bundle branch or fascicular block, can also occur. Treatment for vasospastic angina should include a calcium-channel blocker and/or a nitrate. Vasospastic angina can worsen with use of beta blockers, because they block the vasodilatory effects of beta receptors while leaving vasoconstrictor alpha receptors unblocked.

Pericarditis

The ST segment elevation of pericarditis (Fig. 9.11) has four characteristics that, while not pathognomonic, help to distinguish it from STEACS:

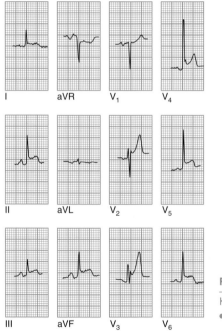

Fig. 9.11 Pericarditis

Key point:
- widespread 'saddle-shaped' ST segment elevation

- The ST segment elevation is typically widespread, affecting all of those leads (anterolateral and inferior) that 'look at' the inflamed epicardium. Leads aVR and V_1 usually show reciprocal ST segment depression.

- The ST segment elevation is characteristically 'saddle shaped' (concave upward).
- T wave inversion occurs only after the ST segments have returned to baseline.
- Q waves do not develop.

The assessment of a patient with pericarditis should aim not only to confirm the diagnosis but also at establishing the cause (Table 9.3).

Table 9.3 Causes of pericarditis

- Infectious
  - viral (e.g. coxsackie)
  - bacterial (e.g. tuberculosis, *Staphylococcus*)
  - fungal
  - parasitic
- Myocardial infarction (first few days)
- Dressler's syndrome (1 month or more post-myocardial infarction)
- Uraemia
- Malignancy
- Connective tissue disease
- Radiotherapy
- Traumatic
- Drug-induced

Clinically, the pain of pericarditis can usually be distinguished from that of myocardial infarction. Although both produce a retrosternal pain, the pain of pericarditis is sharp and pleuritic, exacerbated by inspiration and relieved by sitting forwards. A friction rub on auscultation is pathognomonic of pericarditis.

Direct treatment of the underlying cause should be carried out where possible. Anti-inflammatory agents (e.g. aspirin, indometacin) are often effective. Colchicine can be useful in treating relapsing pericarditis. Systemic corticosteroids can be considered in selected cases, although their role is controversial and they should not be considered without first obtaining specialist advice.

High take-off

Elevation of the ST segment is sometimes seen in the anterior chest leads as a variant of normal, and is referred to as 'high take-off' or 'early repolarization'. A high take-off ST segment always follows an S wave and is not associated with reciprocal ST segment depression; compare its appearances in Figure 9.12 with the earlier ECGs in this chapter.

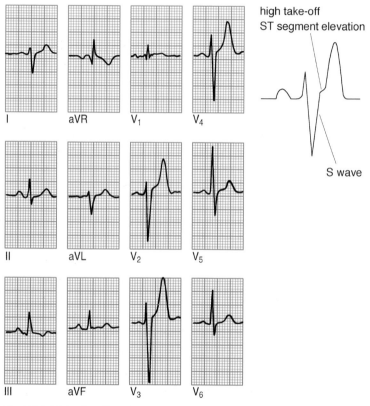

Fig. 9.12 High take-off

Key point: • ST segment elevation follows an S wave

Whenever you suspect ST segment elevation to be just high take-off, always endeavour to find earlier ECGs for confirmation.

Left bundle branch block

Persistent elevation of the ST segment is a feature of the right precordial leads (V_1–V_3) in left bundle branch block. Left bundle branch block is easily identified by the characteristic broadening and notching of the QRS complexes. Left bundle branch block is discussed in more detail in Chapter 8 and is illustrated in Figure 8.11 (p. 149).

● **'Appropriate discordance' in left bundle branch block**
The abnormal pattern of ventricular depolarization in left bundle branch block is followed by an abnormal pattern of repolarization. This manifests itself on the ECG by repolarization (ST segment and T wave) appearances that are discordant with the depolarization (QRS complex) appearances. In other words, where the QRS complex is negative, the following ST segment will be 'positive' (elevated) and the T wave will also be 'positive' (upright). This is known as 'appropriate discordance'.

One useful aspect of this concept is that the presence of *concordance* between the QRS complex and the subsequent ST segment and T wave in the setting of left bundle branch block can be used as an indicator of myocardial ischaemia or infarction. This can be termed 'inappropriate concordance' and applies to ST segment elevation/upright T waves following a positive QRS complex, or ST segment depression/inverted T waves following a negative QRS complex (i.e. in leads V_1–V_3).

Details of a diagnostic scoring system for acute myocardial infarction in the setting of left bundle branch block, based in part on the principle of 'appropriate discordance', can be found in Sgarbossa EB, Pinski SL, Barbagelata A, *et al.* Electrocardiographic diagnosis of evolving acute myocardial infarction in the presence of left bundle-branch block. *New England Journal of Medicine* 1996;**334**:481–7.

Brugada syndrome

The hereditary condition Brugada syndrome, which is caused by an abnormality of the cardiac sodium channel, is characterized on the ECG by right bundle branch block and persistent ST segment elevation in leads V_1–V_3 (Fig. 9.13) and predisposes the patient to syncope and sudden cardiac death secondary to ventricular arrhythmias. It is thought to be responsible for as many as 50 per cent of cases of sudden cardiac death with an 'apparently normal' heart.

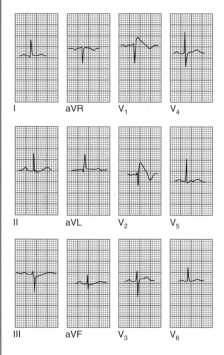

Fig. 9.13 Brugada syndrome

Key points:
- Right bundle branch block
- Anterior ST segment elevation

● Are the ST segments depressed?

Again, look carefully at the ST segment in each lead to see if it is isoelectric (on the same level as the ECG's baseline). If it is below this level, the ST segment is depressed.

If ST segment depression is present, think of the following possible causes:

- myocardial ischaemia
- acute posterior myocardial infarction
- 'reciprocal' changes in ST segment elevation myocardial infarction
- drugs (e.g. digoxin, quinidine)
- ventricular hypertrophy with 'strain'.

If any of these is a possibility, turn to the following pages for guidance on what to do next.

Myocardial ischaemia

Unlike myocardial infarction, ischaemia is reversible and so the associated ECG abnormalities are seen only while the patient is experiencing an episode of pain. ST segment depression is the commonest abnormality associated with ischaemia and is usually 'horizontal' (*cf.* the 'reverse tick' with digoxin effect, p. 180).

Other changes seen in myocardial ischaemia include:

- T wave inversion (Chapter 10)
- T wave 'pseudonormalization' (Chapter 10).

Figure 9.14 shows the ECG of a patient with coronary artery disease during an episode of chest pain.

If myocardial ischaemia is a possibility in your patient, ask about prior episodes of angina and myocardial infarctions. Also ask about risk factors for coronary artery disease (see Table 9.1, p. 162). Stable angina can be assessed further by exercise ECG testing (see Chapter 16).

The management of stable angina includes:

- modifying any risk factors (e.g. smoking, hypertension)
- aspirin, 75 mg once daily
- glyceryl trinitrate sublingually as required
- a statin

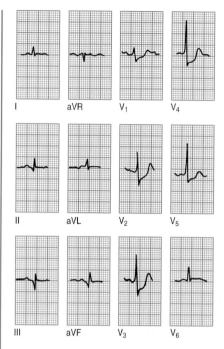

Fig. 9.14 Myocardial ischaemia

Key point:
- anterior ST segment depression with angina

- consideration of an angiotensin-converting enzyme (ACE) inhibitor.

Add anti-anginal treatment as necessary to control symptoms:

- beta blocker
- calcium-channel blocker
- long-acting oral or transdermal or buccal nitrate
- nicorandil
- ivabradine.

If anti-anginal drugs fail to control symptoms adequately, or if non-invasive investigations indicate that the patient is at high risk of an acute coronary syndrome, consider cardiac catheterization with a view to:

- percutaneous coronary intervention
- coronary artery bypass surgery.

Rapidly worsening chest pain, chest pain of recent onset or chest pain at rest in the context of ST segment depression indicate NSTEACS. This is a medical emergency, so urgent treatment is essential. Initial treatment options include:

- bedrest
- analgesia
- aspirin
- clopidogrel
- beta blockers
- intravenous or buccal nitrates
- heparin
- a glycoprotein IIb/IIIa inhibitor.

If an acute coronary syndrome does not settle with drug treatment, consider cardiac catheterization with a view to urgent intervention – discuss this with a cardiologist.

 ACT QUICKLY

Acute coronary syndrome is a medical emergency. Prompt diagnosis and treatment are essential.

Acute posterior myocardial infarction

Acute posterior myocardial infarction is discussed in Chapter 8. It is an ST segment *elevation* myocardial infarction (and the ST segment elevation can be seen if posterior chest leads, V_7–V_9, are recorded), but because the anterior chest leads V_1–V_3 have a reciprocal view of the infarction, these leads show ST segment *depression*, together with:

- dominant R waves
- upright, tall T waves.

An example is shown in Figure 8.4 (p. 141).

The management of acute posterior myocardial infarction is the same of that of other STEMIs, as outlined earlier in this chapter.

ACT QUICKLY

Acute coronary syndrome is a medical emergency. Prompt diagnosis and treatment are essential.

'Reciprocal' changes in ST segment elevation acute coronary syndrome

Just as acute posterior STEMI is associated with ST segment *depression* in the anterior chest leads (V_1–V_3), so any other STEACS can be associated with ST segment depression in leads that are 'distant' from the actual site of the myocardial event (Fig. 9.6, p. 166).

This phenomenon is seen in 30 per cent of anterior STEACS and up to 80 per cent of inferior myocardial STEACS, and the presence of reciprocal ST segment depression can be a useful pointer towards a diagnosis of STEACS where the implication of ST segment elevation is uncertain.

Although such ECG changes have traditionally been considered 'reciprocal' (i.e. a mirror image of electrical changes in the myocardium affected), there is some evidence that the ST segment depression is actually the result of ischaemia in a myocardial territory distant from the infarction site. The presence of 'reciprocal' ST segment depression in the context of STEACS is associated with more extensive coronary disease and carries a worse prognosis.

Drugs

Two anti-arrhythmic drugs affect the ST segment:

- digoxin
- quinidine.

Digoxin has a characteristic effect on the ST segment, which is just one of its many effects on the whole ECG (Table 9.4). The ST segment depression seen with digoxin is described as a 'reverse tick' and is most obvious in leads with tall R waves (Fig. 9.15).

Table 9.4 Effects of digoxin on the ECG

At therapeutic levels
- ST segment depression ('reverse tick')
- Reduction in T wave size
- Shortening of the QT interval

At toxic levels
- T wave inversion
- Arrhythmias – almost any, but especially:
  - sinus bradycardia
  - paroxysmal atrial tachycardia with block
  - atrioventricular block
  - ventricular ectopics
  - ventricular bigeminy
  - ventricular tachycardia

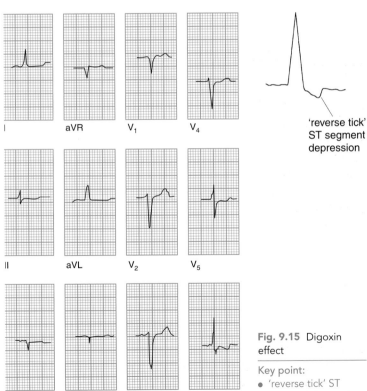

'reverse tick' ST segment depression

Fig. 9.15 Digoxin effect

Key point:
- 'reverse tick' ST segment depression

You must always distinguish between digoxin effects, which may be apparent at therapeutic doses, and digoxin toxicity, which indicates overdosage. If digoxin toxicity is a possibility, ask about symptoms (anorexia, nausea, vomiting, abdominal pain and visual disturbance) and check the patient's digoxin and plasma potassium levels (arrhythmias are more likely if the patient is hypokalaemic).

Treat digoxin toxicity by stopping the drug and, where necessary, correcting potassium levels and treating arrhythmias. A digoxin-specific antibody may be used if the problem is life-threatening, but not without expert advice.

Quinidine also has a number of effects on the ECG, one of which is ST segment depression (which is not 'reverse tick' in character).

DRUG POINT

A complete drug history is essential in any patient with an abnormal ECG.

Ventricular hypertrophy with 'strain'

The appearances of both left and right ventricular hypertrophy are discussed in Chapter 8. The 'strain' pattern is said to be present when, in addition to tall R waves and deep S waves, there is also:

- ST segment depression
- T wave inversion

in the leads that 'look at' the affected ventricle (Fig. 9.16).

The term 'strain' is rather misleading, because the underlying mechanism is unclear. If you see T wave inversion in the presence of other ECG evidence of ventricular hypertrophy, assess the patient carefully as described in Chapter 8, both for further evidence of ventricular hypertrophy and for an underlying cause.

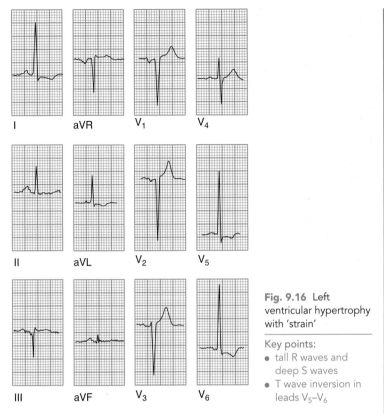

Fig. 9.16 Left ventricular hypertrophy with 'strain'

Key points:
- tall R waves and deep S waves
- T wave inversion in leads V_5–V_6

Are J waves present?

J waves, also known as Osborn waves, are typically seen in hypothermia (below 33°C). J waves have been reported to be present in around 80 per cent of ECGs in hypothermic patients, but they are also sometimes seen in patients with a normal body temperature and are therefore not completely specific for hypothermia.

The J wave is a small positive deflection at the junction between the QRS complex and the ST segment (Fig. 9.17) and is usually best seen in the inferior limb leads and the lateral chest leads.

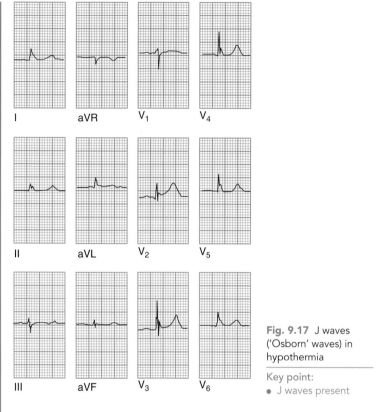

I aVR V₁ V₄

II aVL V₂ V₅

III aVF V₃ V₆

Fig. 9.17 J waves ('Osborn' waves) in hypothermia

Key point:
- J waves present

Patients with hypothermia may also exhibit other ECG abnormalities, including AV block, atrial fibrillation, broadening of the QRS complexes, prolongation of the QT interval, ventricular arrhythmias and asystole.

Summary

To assess the ST segment, ask the following questions:

1. Are the ST segments elevated?

If 'yes', consider:

- ST segment elevation acute coronary syndrome
- left ventricular aneurysm
- Prinzmetal's (vasospastic) angina
- pericarditis
- high take-off
- left bundle branch block
- Brugada syndrome.

2 Are the ST segments depressed?

If 'yes', consider:

- myocardial ischaemia
- acute posterior myocardial infarction
- 'reciprocal' changes in ST segment elevation myocardial infarction
- drugs (digoxin, quinidine)
- ventricular hypertrophy with 'strain'.

3 Are J waves present?

If 'yes', consider:

- hypothermia.

The T wave

After examining the ST segment, look carefully at the size and orientation of the T wave. The T wave corresponds to ventricular repolarization. The shape and orientation of normal T waves are shown in Figure 10.1.

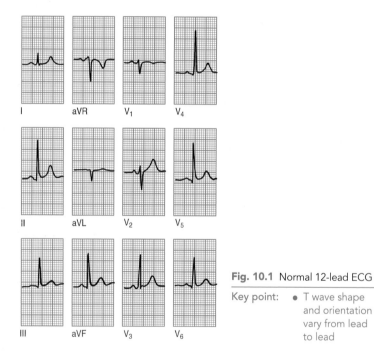

Fig. 10.1 Normal 12-lead ECG

Key point: • T wave shape
             and orientation
             vary from lead
             to lead

It is normal for the T wave to be inverted in leads V_1 and aVR. In some cases, T wave inversion can also be normal in leads

III and V$_2$, and sometimes even V$_3$, and these occurrences are discussed later in this chapter.

T waves can be abnormal in one of three ways, so the questions you need to ask about them are:

- Are the T waves too tall?
- Are the T waves too small?
- Are any of the T waves inverted?

● Are the T waves too tall?

There is no clearly defined normal range for T wave height, although, as a general guide, a T wave should be no more than half the size of the preceding QRS complex. Your ability to recognize abnormally tall T waves will improve as you examine increasing numbers of ECGs and gain experience of the normal variations that occur.

If you suspect that the T waves are abnormally tall, consider whether your patient could have either of the following:

- hyperkalaemia
- acute coronary syndrome.

If either is a possibility, turn to the following pages for guidance on what to do next.

Bear in mind, however, that tall T waves are often just a variant of normal, especially if you are judging just a single ECG. Your level of suspicion should be higher if you are comparing against earlier ECGs from the same patient and the height of the T waves has increased considerably.

Hyperkalaemia

An elevated plasma potassium level can cause tall 'tented' T waves (Fig. 10.2).

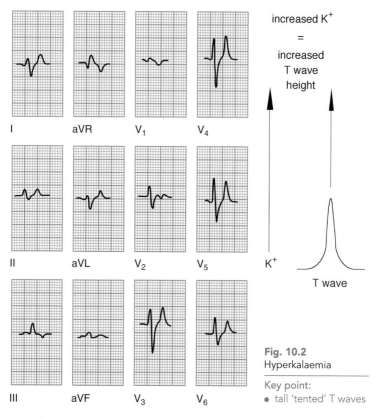

increased K⁺
=
increased
T wave
height

K⁺

T wave

Fig. 10.2
Hyperkalaemia

Key point:
● tall 'tented' T waves

Hyperkalaemia may also widen the T waves so that the entire ST segment is incorporated into the upstroke of the T wave. Hyperkalaemia may also cause:

● flattening and even loss of the P wave
● lengthening of the PR interval
● widening of the QRS complex
● arrhythmias.

If the diagnosis is confirmed by a raised plasma potassium level, assess the patient for symptoms and signs of an underlying cause (e.g. renal failure). In particular, review their treatment chart for inappropriate potassium supplements and potassium-sparing diuretics.

DRUG POINT

A complete drug history is essential in any patient with an abnormal ECG.

Because of the risk of fatal cardiac arrhythmias, hyperkalaemia needs urgent treatment if it is causing ECG abnormalities or the plasma potassium level is above 6.5 mmol/L.

ACT QUICKLY

Severe hyperkalaemia is a medical emergency. Prompt diagnosis and treatment are essential.

Acute coronary syndrome

Tall 'hyperacute' T waves may be seen in the early stages of an acute coronary syndrome (Fig. 10.3). Increased T wave height may be a result of potassium released from damaged myocytes, leading to a localized hyperkalaemia.

Tall T waves are particularly characteristic of acute posterior myocardial infarction (p. 139). Infarction of the posterior wall of the left ventricle leads to reciprocal (i.e. 'mirror-image') changes when viewed from the perspective of the anterior chest leads. Thus, the usual myocardial infarction appearances of pathological Q waves, ST segment elevation and inverted T waves will appear as R waves, ST segment depression and upright, tall T waves when viewed from leads V_1–V_3 (see Fig. 8.4).

The diagnosis and management of acute coronary syndrome are discussed in detail in Chapter 9.

SEEK HELP

Acute myocardial infarction requires urgent treatment. Obtain the advice of a cardiologist without delay.

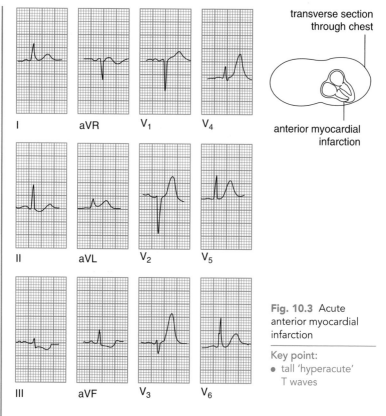

transverse section
through chest

anterior myocardial
infarction

Fig. 10.3 Acute
anterior myocardial
infarction

Key point:
- tall 'hyperacute'
  T waves

I aVR V₁ V₄

II aVL V₂ V₅

III aVF V₃ V₆

● Are the T waves too small?

As with tall T waves, the judgement of whether T waves are
abnormally small is subjective.

If you suspect that the T waves are abnormally small, consider
whether your patient could have one of the following:

- hypokalaemia
- pericardial effusion
- hypothyroidism.

Advice about the diagnosis and treatment of each of these is
given below.

Hypokalaemia

Just as hyperkalaemia causes tall T waves, so hypokalaemia causes small T waves (Fig. 10.4).

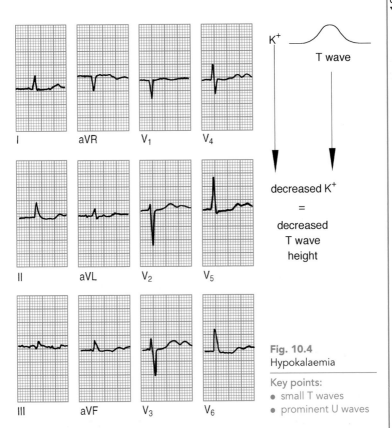

Fig. 10.4
Hypokalaemia

Key points:
- small T waves
- prominent U waves

Look carefully for other ECG changes that may accompany hypokalaemia:

- first-degree heart block
- depression of the ST segment
- prominent U waves.

If hypokalaemia is suspected, assess the patient for symptoms (e.g. muscle weakness, cramps) and review the treatment chart. Although many conditions lead to hypokalaemia, the commonest cause is diuretics.

DRUG POINT

A complete drug history is essential in any patient with an abnormal ECG.

More severe hypokalaemia, or the presence of symptoms, requires cautious correction with a slow intravenous infusion of potassium chloride.

ACT QUICKLY

Severe hypokalaemia is a medical emergency. Prompt diagnosis and treatment are essential.

Pericardial effusion

If the whole ECG, and not just the T waves, is of a low voltage, think about the possibility of pericardial effusion.

For a detailed discussion of the investigation and treatment of pericardial effusion, see p. 144.

Hypothyroidism

Hypothyroidism can cause small QRS complexes and small T waves, but the most characteristic finding is sinus bradycardia (p. 31).

Perform a careful history and examination, and confirm the diagnosis with T_3, T_4 and thyroid-stimulating hormone levels.

● Are any of the T waves inverted?

If T wave inversion is present, begin by asking:

● Could this be normal?

T wave inversion is considered normal in:

● leads aVR and V_1 (see Fig. 10.1)
● lead V_2 in younger people
● lead V_3 in black people (Fig. 10.5).

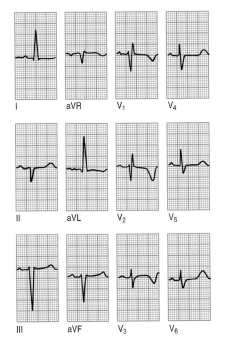

| I | aVR | V_1 | V_4 |

| II | aVL | V_2 | V_5 |

| III | aVF | V_3 | V_6 |

Fig. 10.5 T wave inversion in a normal black person

Key point:
● T wave inversion can be normal in leads V_1–V_3 in black people

T wave inversion in lead III can also be normal, and may be accompanied by a small Q wave – both of these findings can disappear if the ECG is repeated with the patient's breath held in deep inspiration (see Fig. 7.3, p. 129).

T wave inversion in any other lead is generally considered abnormal, and if it is present, consider whether your patient has one of the following:

- myocardial ischaemia
- myocardial infarction
- ventricular hypertrophy with 'strain'
- digoxin toxicity.

You will find advice about the recognition and management of each of these conditions below.

There are also several conditions in which T wave inversion occurs in combination with other ECG abnormalities. If the ECG has been normal up to this point of the assessment, it is unlikely that any of the following are to blame for the T wave inversion. Nonetheless, if you still have not found a cause after going through the list above, consider:

- repolarization abnormalities following a paroxysmal tachycardia (Chapter 3)
- bundle branch block (Chapter 8)
- pericarditis (Chapter 9)
- permanent ventricular pacing (Chapter 14).

Finally, there are four conditions in which T wave inversion can occur but the ECG is not diagnostic:

- hyperventilation
- mitral valve prolapse
- pulmonary embolism
- subarachnoid haemorrhage.

If your patient has one of these conditions, you do not need to look for another cause of T wave inversion unless there are other reasons to suspect one.

Myocardial ischaemia

ST segment depression is the commonest manifestation of myocardial ischaemia (Chapter 9), but T wave inversion may also occur in the leads that 'look at' the affected areas (Fig. 10.6). Because ischaemia is reversible, these ECG abnormalities will only be observed during an ischaemic episode.

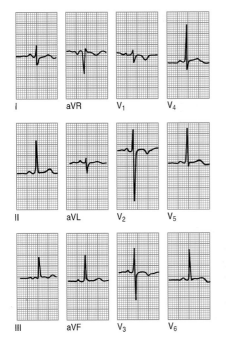

I   aVR   V₁   V₄

II   aVL   V₂   V₅

III   aVF   V₃   V₆

Fig. 10.6 T wave inversion with myocardial ischaemia

Key point:
- reversible T wave inversion (leads V_1–V_3) with myocardial ischaemia

Patients whose T waves are inverted to begin with (e.g. following a myocardial infarction) may develop temporarily upright T waves during ischaemic episodes. This is referred to as T wave 'pseudonormalization'.

The management of myocardial ischaemia is described in detail on page 177.

Myocardial infarction

T wave inversion can occur not only as a temporary change in myocardial ischaemia but also as a more prolonged (and sometimes permanent) change in myocardial infarction. In Chapter 9, we mentioned that myocardial infarctions are often divided into:

- ST segment elevation myocardial infarction (STEMI)
- non-ST segment elevation myocardial infarction (NSTEMI).

T wave inversion can occur in either type of infarct. In STEMI, the T wave inversion accompanies the return of the elevated ST segment to baseline (Fig. 10.7). T wave inversion may be

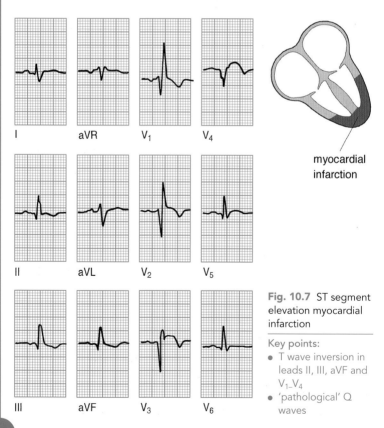

I aVR V$_1$ V$_4$

II aVL V$_2$ V$_5$

III aVF V$_3$ V$_6$

myocardial infarction

Fig. 10.7 ST segment elevation myocardial infarction

Key points:
- T wave inversion in leads II, III, aVF and V$_1$-V$_4$
- 'pathological' Q waves

permanent, or the T wave may return to normal. NSTEMI also causes T wave inversion, although it can also manifest as ST segment depression alone.

If you see abnormal T wave inversion on an ECG, question the patient about any history of chest pain and previous angina or myocardial infarctions and assess their risk factors for ischaemic heart disease (see Table 9.1, p. 162).

The management of acute coronary syndrome is detailed in Chapter 9.

> **ACT QUICKLY**
>
> Acute coronary syndrome is a medical emergency. Prompt diagnosis and treatment are essential.

Ventricular hypertrophy

In addition to tall R waves and deep S waves (Chapter 8), ventricular hypertrophy can also cause ST segment depression and T wave inversion. This is commonly referred to as a 'strain' pattern (p. 182).

If present, the 'strain' pattern is seen in the leads that 'look at' the hypertrophied ventricle. With left ventricular hypertrophy the abnormalities will be seen in leads I, aVL and V_4–V_6. Right ventricular hypertrophy causes changes in leads V_1–V_3.

The term 'strain' is rather misleading because the underlying mechanism is unclear. Although some conditions, such as massive pulmonary embolism, can certainly place a ventricle under an increased workload and are associated with the 'strain' pattern, it is also seen in cases of ventricular hypertrophy where there is no apparent stress on the ventricle.

If you see T wave inversion in the presence of other ECG evidence of ventricular hypertrophy, assess the patient carefully as described in Chapter 8.

Digoxin toxicity

Always check if a patient with T wave inversion is receiving treatment with digoxin, as this can be an indication of digoxin toxicity (Fig. 10.8). This is just one of a number of ECG changes that can be seen in patients taking digoxin (see Table 9.4, p. 181).

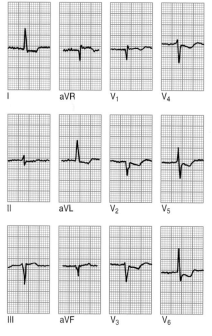

Fig. 10.8 Digoxin toxicity

Key points:
- T wave inversion in leads V_2–V_6
- patient on digoxin for atrial fibrillation

The diagnosis and treatment of digoxin toxicity are covered in more detail on page 180.

DRUG POINT

A complete drug history is essential in any patient with an abnormal ECG.

Summary

To assess the T wave, ask the following questions:

1. Are the T waves too tall?

If 'yes', consider:

- hyperkalaemia
- acute myocardial infarction.

2. Are the T waves too small?

If 'yes', consider:

- hypokalaemia
- pericardial effusion
- hypothyroidism.

3. Are any of the T waves inverted?

If 'yes', consider:

- normal (leads aVR and V_1)
- normal variant (leads V_2, V_3 and III)
- myocardial ischaemia
- myocardial infarction
- ventricular hypertrophy with 'strain'
- digoxin toxicity.

Also bear in mind:

- repolarization abnormalities following a paroxysmal tachycardia (Chapter 3)

- bundle branch block (Chapter 8)
- pericarditis (Chapter 9)
- permanent ventricular pacing (Chapter 14)
- hyperventilation
- mitral valve prolapse
- pulmonary embolism
- subarachnoid haemorrhage.

11 The QT interval

After examining the T waves, measure the QT interval. This is the time from the *start* of the QRS complex to the *end* of the T wave (Fig. 11.1), and it represents the total duration of electrical activity (depolarization and repolarization) in the ventricles.

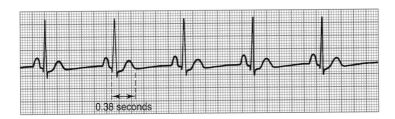

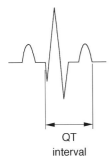

QT interval

Fig. 11.1 The QT interval

Key point: • QT interval is 0.38 s in this patient

When determining the duration of the QT interval, it is important to measure it to the end of the T wave and not the U wave (if one is present – see Chapter 12). It is easy to mistake a

U wave for a T wave and thus overestimate the QT interval. To reduce the likelihood of this, measure the QT interval in lead aVL, in which U waves are least prominent.

As with any interval in the ECG, there are only two possible abnormalities of the QT interval:

- The QT interval can be too long.
- The QT interval can be too short.

Unfortunately, deciding whether or not the QT interval is normal is not entirely straightforward, because the duration varies according to the patient's heart rate: the faster the heart rate, the shorter the QT interval. To allow for this, you must calculate the corrected QT interval (QT_c) using the following formula:

$$QT_c = \frac{QT}{\sqrt{RR}}$$

where QT_c is the corrected QT interval, QT is the measured QT interval and RR is the measured RR interval (all measurements in seconds).

If you are interested in the theory behind QT interval correction, see the box opposite.

A normal QT_c interval is 0.35–0.44 s long. However, it is worth noting that there is not an absolutely clear cut-off between normal and abnormal at 0.44 s, and results just on either side of this value could be regarded as borderline. Furthermore, QT intervals tend to be a little longer in women than in men, so some authorities quote the normal upper limit of the QT_c interval as 0.44 s in men and 0.45 s in women.

When you assess the QT interval, therefore, ask yourself the following two questions:

- Is the QT_c interval shorter than 0.35 s?
- Is the QT_c interval longer than 0.44 s?

If the answer to either question is 'yes', turn to the relevant section of this chapter to find out what to do next. If 'no', you can move on to the next chapter.

● Why correct the QT interval?

Correction of the QT interval is necessary because the normal QT interval varies with heart rate: the faster the heart rate, the shorter the normal QT interval. Although graphs and tables of normal QT intervals at different heart rates are available, it is inconvenient to have to look up the normal range every time you want to check someone's QT interval.

A much better way to assess a QT interval is to correct it to what it *would* be if the patient's heart rate was 60 beats/min. By doing this, all you will then need to remember is *one* normal range for the QT interval.

You will need a pocket calculator to calculate the corrected QT interval ('QT_c interval'). Divide the patient's measured QT interval (measured in seconds) by the square root of their RR interval (also measured in seconds). This is Bazett's formula:

$$QT_c = \frac{QT}{\sqrt{RR}}$$

The RR interval is the time between consecutive R waves, and can be either measured directly from the ECG or calculated by dividing 60 by the patient's heart rate. For example, at a heart rate of 80 beats/min the RR interval is 0.75 s.

Many of the more sophisticated ECG machines automatically print out a value for the QT_c interval on the ECG. However, always check for yourself values that are automatically measured in this way, as errors do occur.

The normal range for the QT interval at a heart rate of 60 beats/min, and thus for the QT_c interval, is 0.35–0.44 s.

● Is the QT$_c$ interval shorter than 0.35 s?

If the answer is 'yes', the patient's corrected QT interval is shorter than normal and you should check for the following:

● congenital short QT syndromes
● hypercalcaemia
● digoxin effect.

If either of these is a possibility, read below to find out what to do next.

Shortening of the QT$_c$ interval is also recognized in hyperthermia.

Having established the diagnosis of hyperthermia clinically, you will not need to look for another cause for a shortened QT$_c$ interval unless there is a good reason to do so.

Congenital short QT syndromes

Although congenital long QT syndromes are well recognized, it is only in the past few years that congenital short QT syndromes have been clearly described. The congenital short QT syndromes appear to follow an autosomal dominant pattern of inheritance and mutations affecting the genes *KCNH2*, *KCNQ1* and *KCNJ2* (which are linked to different potassium channels) have been identified. Most patients have inducible ventricular fibrillation on electrophysiological testing and a family history of sudden cardiac death or atrial fibrillation. The QT$_c$ interval is usually very short indeed, and the diagnosis should be certainly considered on finding a QT$_c$ interval below 0.33 s.

Implantation of a cardioverter defibrillator forms the cornerstone of treatment, although this can be challenging in view of the very young age at which the condition is diagnosed in some individuals. Drug treatment to lengthen the QT interval may be possible, depending upon the subtype of short QT syndrome. The management of this condition is complex and requires the input of a cardiologist with a special interest in arrhythmias.

Hypercalcaemia

The shortened QT interval in hypercalcaemia results from abnormally rapid ventricular repolarization (Fig. 11.2).

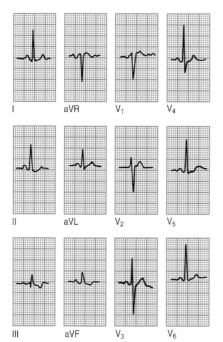

I   aVR   V₁   V₄

II   aVL   V₂   V₅

III   aVF   V₃   V₆

Fig. 11.2 Short QT interval in hypercalcaemia

Key points:
- QT interval is 0.26 s
- heart rate is 100 beats/min, QT_c interval is 0.34 s

Symptoms of hypercalcaemia include anorexia, weight loss, nausea, vomiting, abdominal pain, constipation, polydipsia, polyuria, weakness and depression.

A prominent U wave may also be seen in hypercalcaemia. Confirm the diagnosis with a plasma calcium level (correcting the result for the patient's current albumin level). The underlying causes that you need to consider are listed in Table 11.1.

Table 11.1 Causes of hypercalcaemia

- Hyperparathyroidism
  - primary
  - tertiary
- Malignancy (including myeloma)
- Drugs
  - thiazide diuretics
  - excessive vitamin D intake
- Sarcoidosis
- Thyrotoxicosis
- Milk-alkali syndrome

The treatment of hypercalcaemia depends, in the long term, on the underlying cause. Immediate management depends on the symptoms and plasma calcium level. There is a risk of cardiac arrest with severe hypercalcaemia, so prompt recognition and treatment are essential.

Severe symptoms (e.g. vomiting, drowsiness) or a plasma calcium level greater than 3.5 mmol/L warrant urgent treatment as follows:

- intravenous 0.9 per cent saline (e.g. 3–4 L/24 h)
- intravenous furosemide (20–40 mg every 6–12 h *after rehydration*)
- bisphosphonates (e.g. disodium pamidronate – single infusion of 30 mg over 2 h)
- discontinuation of thiazides/vitamin D compounds
- monitoring of urea and electrolytes and calcium levels every 12 h.

 ACT QUICKLY

Severe hypercalcaemia is a medical emergency. Prompt diagnosis and treatment are essential.

Digoxin effect

Shortening of the QT interval is one of several effects that treatment with digoxin has on the ECG (see Table 9.4, p. 181).

It is important to note that digoxin *effects* are normal, and do not imply that the patient has digoxin *toxicity*. The effects of digoxin on the ECG are covered in more detail in Chapter 9.

DRUG POINT

A complete drug history is essential in any patient with an abnormal ECG.

● Is the QT$_c$ interval longer than 0.44 s?

If the answer is 'yes', the patient's corrected QT interval is prolonged (although remember that QT intervals tend to be a little longer in women, so some authorities quote the normal upper limit as 0.45 s in women).

The causes you need to consider are:

- hypocalcaemia
- drug effects
- acute myocarditis
- long QT syndrome.

If any of these is a possibility, consult the following pages to find out what to do next.

In addition, there are also several conditions in which QT interval prolongation is recognized, but in which this abnormality is an interesting feature rather than a useful diagnostic pointer. Such conditions include:

- acute myocardial infarction
- cerebral injury
- hypertrophic cardiomyopathy
- hypothermia.

You simply need to be aware that QT interval prolongation is recognized in these conditions, so that you do not need to look for another cause unless clinically suspected.

Hypocalcaemia

Hypocalcaemia is a well-recognized cause of QT interval prolongation (Fig. 11.3).

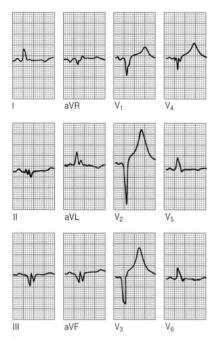

Fig. 11.3 Long QT interval in hypocalcaemia

Key points:
- QT interval is 0.57 s
- heart rate is 51 beats/min, QT_c interval is 0.52 s

The clinical features (peripheral and circumoral paraesthesiae, tetany, fits and psychiatric disturbance) are characteristic. Look for Trousseau's sign (carpal spasm when the brachial artery is occluded with a blood-pressure cuff), Chvostek's sign (twitching of facial muscles when tapping over the facial nerve) and papilloedema. Confirm the diagnosis by checking a plasma calcium level on an uncuffed blood sample, not forgetting to check a simultaneous albumin level so that any necessary correction can be made.

Once a diagnosis of hypocalcaemia has been made, always look for the underlying cause (Table 11.2).

Table 11.2 Causes of hypocalcaemia

- Hypoparathyroidism
  - following thyroid surgery
  - autoimmune
  - congenital (DiGeorge's syndrome)
- Pseudohypoparathyroidism
- Chronic renal failure
- Vitamin D deficiency/resistance
- Drugs (e.g. calcitonin)
- Acute pancreatitis

The treatment of hypocalcaemia depends on the severity of symptoms. Treat severe hypocalcaemia with intravenous calcium (given as 10 mL calcium gluconate 10 per cent). Treat those who have milder symptoms with oral calcium supplements and, if necessary, oral vitamin D derivatives. Carefully monitor plasma calcium levels to avoid over-treatment and consequent hypercalcaemia.

Drug effects

Several anti-arrhythmic drugs cause prolongation of the QT interval by slowing myocardial conduction, and thus repolarization. Examples are quinidine, procainamide and flecainide. QT interval prolongation is also seen with terfenadine and tricyclic antidepressants.

Drug-induced QT interval prolongation is associated with torsades de pointes (Chapter 3), which can lead to ventricular fibrillation and sudden cardiac death. The problem therefore requires immediate attention, and referral to a cardiologist for review of anti-arrhythmic drug treatment is recommended.

DRUG POINT

A complete drug history is essential in any patient with an abnormal ECG.

Acute myocarditis

QT interval prolongation can occur with any cause of acute myocarditis, although it is usually associated with rheumatic carditis.

Presenting features often include a fever, chest discomfort, palpitations and symptoms of heart failure (dyspnoea and fatigue). Examination may reveal quiet heart sounds, a friction rub, tachycardia, a fourth heart sound and gallop rhythm. There may also be features specific to the underlying cause (Table 11.3).

Table 11.3 Causes of myocarditis

- Infectious
  - viral (e.g. coxsackie, influenza)
  - bacterial (e.g. acute rheumatic fever, diphtheria)
  - protozoal (e.g. Chagas' disease, toxoplasmosis)
  - rickettsial
- Drug induced (e.g. chloroquine)
- Toxic agents (e.g. lead)
- Peripartum

Other ECG changes may be present, including:

- ST segment changes
- T wave inversion
- heart block (of any degree of severity)
- arrhythmias.

A chest radiograph may show cardiomegaly. A cardiac biopsy reveals acute inflammatory changes, and the levels of cardiac enzymes will be raised. Rarely, viral serology may establish the aetiology.

The treatment of acute myocarditis is supportive. Bedrest is recommended. Treat heart failure, arrhythmias and heart block as necessary. Antibiotics are indicated where a responsive organism is suspected. Although many patients will go on to make a good recovery, some are left with heart failure.

SEEK HELP

Acute myocarditis requires specialist assessment. Obtain the advice of a cardiologist without delay.

Long QT syndrome

Many hereditary syndromes are now recognized in which an abnormality of the sodium or potassium ion channels causes a susceptibility to ventricular arrhythmias and sudden cardiac death. These syndromes include **long QT syndrome** (LQTS), in which genetic abnormalities of the potassium or sodium channels lead to prolonged ventricular repolarization and hence prolongation of the QT interval.

Several genetic abnormalities have now been identified, the three most common being termed LQT1 and LQT2 (potassium channel abnormalities) and LQT3 (sodium channel abnormality). The classification of LQTS includes the hereditary syndromes:

● Romano–Ward syndrome
● Jervell and Lange-Nielsen syndrome.

The autosomal dominant Romano–Ward syndrome consists of recurrent syncopal attacks and sudden death secondary to ventricular tachycardia, torsades de pointes and ventricular fibrillation. The arrhythmias are often triggered by exercise or stress.

The autosomal recessive Jervell and Lange-Nielsen syndrome is much rarer and carries the same risk of ventricular arrhythmias. Unlike the Romano–Ward syndrome, it is also associated with congenital high-tone deafness.

Patients with long QT syndrome need careful risk assessment and will usually require anti-arrhythmic medication. Those at high risk of ventricular arrhythmias will usually need an implantable cardioverter defibrillator.

 SEEK HELP

Long QT syndrome is potentially life-threatening. Obtain the advice of a cardiologist without delay.

Summary

To assess the QT interval, ask the following questions:

1. Is the QT_c interval shorter than 0.35 s?

If 'yes', consider:

- hereditary short QT syndromes
- hypercalcaemia
- digoxin effect (p. 180).

Also bear in mind:

- hyperthermia.

2. Is the QT_c interval longer than 0.44 s?

If 'yes', consider:

- hypocalcaemia
- drug effects
- acute myocarditis
- long QT syndrome.

Also bear in mind:

- acute myocardial infarction (p. 159)
- cerebral injury
- hypertrophic cardiomyopathy
- hypothermia.

12 The U wave

The U wave follows the T wave (Fig. 12.1) and is commonly seen in normal ECGs, although it can be difficult to discern clearly. When present, U waves are most clearly seen in the anterior chest leads V_2-V_4.

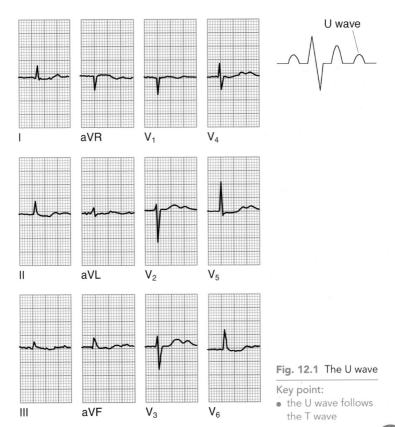

Fig. 12.1 The U wave

Key point:
- the U wave follows the T wave

Although it is suggested that the U wave is caused by repolarization of the interventricular septum, this is by no means certain.

Normally, U waves are small and point in the same direction as the preceding T wave. Therefore, inverted U waves usually follow inverted T waves, and result from the same clinical abnormality (see Chapter 10).

U waves can also be abnormal in their own right, so when you assess the U wave, ask the following question:

● Do the U waves appear too prominent?

If the answer is 'yes', you will find a list of causes to consider in the next section.

● Do the U waves appear too prominent?

This is not a straightforward question to answer, because there is no normal range that you can apply to the height of a U wave. Suspecting the U waves are too prominent therefore depends on subjective judgement rather than an objective measurement, and there is no substitute for reporting large numbers of ECGs to gain experience of the range of normality of the U wave (and, for that matter, all other aspects of the ECG).

It follows on from this that you should not attach too much weight to U wave prominence. Simply regard it as a clue that your patient may have one of the following:

● hypokalaemia
● hypercalcaemia
● hyperthyroidism.

If any of these is a possibility, turn to the appropriate section of this chapter to find out what to do next.

Hypokalaemia

Prominent U waves can be just one of a number of ECG abnormalities seen in the hypokalaemic patient (Fig. 12.2). Other associated ECG changes include:

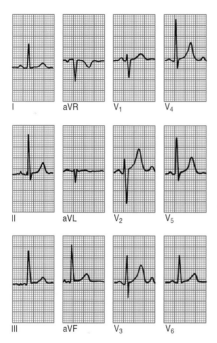

Fig. 12.2 Hypokalaemia

Key point:
● prominent U waves in leads V$_2$–V$_4$

● first-degree atrioventricular block (Chapter 6)
● depression of the ST segment (Chapter 9)
● small T waves (Chapter 10).

The investigation and treatment of hypokalaemia are discussed in detail on page 191.

ACT QUICKLY

Severe hypokalaemia is a medical emergency. Prompt diagnosis and treatment are essential.

Hypercalcaemia

Always think of hypercalcaemia if you see prominent U waves, although hypercalcaemia is more characteristically associated with shortening of the QT interval (Chapter 11).

Confirm the diagnosis with a plasma calcium level (correcting the result for the patient's current albumin level).

The management of hypercalcaemia is discussed in detail on page 205.

Hyperthyroidism

Prominent U waves in association with a tachycardia (Chapter 2) should prompt you to think of hyperthyroidism, although the U wave abnormality is not commonly seen in this condition.

Confirm the diagnosis with T_3, T_4 and thyroid-stimulating hormone levels.

Summary

To assess the U wave, ask the following question:

1. *Do the U waves appear too prominent?*

If 'yes', consider:

- hypokalaemia
- hypercalcaemia
- hyperthyroidism.

Note. U waves can also be inverted, but this usually accompanies T wave inversion, the causes of which are discussed in Chapter 10.

13 Artefacts on the ECG

If you encounter ECG abnormalities that appear atypical or that do not fit with the patient's clinical condition, always consider the possibility that they may be artefacts caused by:

- electrode misplacement
- external electrical interference
- incorrect calibration
- incorrect paper speed
- patient movement.

Examples of each of these are discussed on the following pages.

- Remember
  - Never give undue weight to a single investigation, particularly if the result does not fit with your clinical findings.
  - Do not hesitate to repeat an ECG if you suspect that the abnormalities could be artefacts.

● Electrode misplacement

The correct position of each recording electrode is given in Chapter 1. It can be quite easy to swap two electrodes inadvertently; this is particularly common with the limb electrodes.

Figure 13.1 shows an ECG recorded with the two arm electrodes swapped over. The abnormalities can be quite subtle, but you should always think of electrode misplacement if you see unexpected wave inversions.

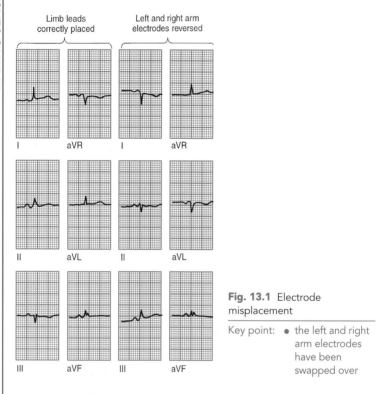

Fig. 13.1 Electrode misplacement

Key point: • the left and right arm electrodes have been swapped over

● External electrical interference

External electrical interference (e.g. from electrical appliances) seldom causes difficulties when recording ECGs in hospital. However, for general practitioners who sometimes record ECGs in patients' homes, 50 Hz electrical interference from domestic appliances has been reported as a major cause of ECG artefact, and this can make the ECG difficult or even impossible to interpret correctly.

Always bear this in mind when interpreting an ECG recorded in a patient's home. Unless the source of the interference can be identified and removed, there is little that can be done apart from repeating the recording with the patient in a new location.

● Incorrect calibration

The standard ECG is recorded so that a voltage of 1 mV makes the recording needle move 10 mm (1 cm). Every ECG must include a calibration mark (Fig. 13.2) so that the gain setting can be checked. If you see waves that appear too big or too small, always double-check the size of the calibration mark (Fig. 13.3).

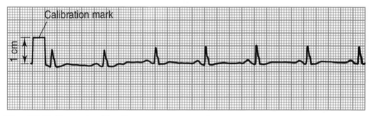

Fig. 13.2 Correct calibration

Key points: ● note the 1 cm calibration mark
● 1 mV = 1 cm

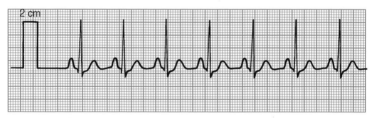

Fig. 13.3 Incorrect calibration

Key point: ● 1 mV = 2 cm

Sometimes it is necessary to alter the gain setting, particularly if the QRS complexes are so big at the standard setting that they will not fit clearly on the paper. If it is necessary to change to a non-standard calibration, it is good practice to record this clearly by writing a note on the ECG.

● Incorrect paper speed

In the UK and USA, the standard ECG recording speed is 25 mm/s, so that 1 small (1 mm) square equals 0.04 s. If the paper is run at double the speed (50 mm/s, which is standard in some parts of Europe), the waves will double in width (Fig. 13.4). Always label every ECG you record with the paper speed used and, if you use a non-standard setting, it is good practice to document this clearly at the top of the ECG.

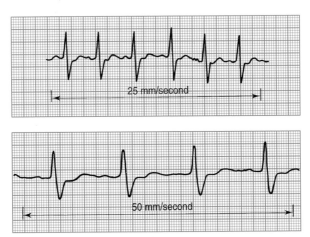

25 mm/second

50 mm/second

Fig. 13.4 Paper speed and wave width

Key point: ● waves are wider at higher paper speeds

● Patient movement

The ECG records the electrical activity of the heart, but this is not the only source of electrical activity in the body. Skeletal muscle activity is also picked up on the ECG, and it is important for patients to lie still and relaxed while an ECG is being recorded. Unfortunately, this is not always possible, particularly if the patient:

● is uncooperative or agitated
● is in respiratory distress
● has a movement disorder.

Skeletal muscle activity is unavoidable during exercise testing. The use of signal-averaged ECGs, which 'average out' random electrical artefacts by combining a number of PQRST complexes, can help (Fig. 13.5). However, signal-averaged recordings can also be misleading by introducing artefactual changes of their own, and such recordings should always be interpreted with discretion.

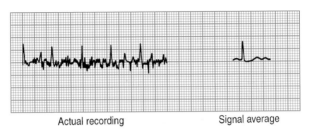

Actual recording   Signal average

Fig. 13.5 Signal-averaged ECG

Key point: ● electrical artefacts are reduced by signal averaging

Summary

For any ECG abnormality, always ask yourself:

1. Could this be artefactual?

If 'yes', consider:

● electrode misplacement
● external electrical interference
● incorrect calibration
● incorrect paper speed
● patient movement.

Pacemakers and implantable cardioverter defibrillators

14

It is beyond the scope of this handbook to provide a detailed discussion of pacemakers and automatic implantable cardioverter defibrillators (ICDs). However, we have included a brief overview in this chapter for two reasons:

- Pacemakers and ICDs are effective treatments for several of the problems described in this book.
- Pacing affects the appearance of the ECG.

On the following pages you will find a general description of what pacemakers and ICDs do, along with their indications.

● What do pacemakers do?

Rapid advances in pacemaker technology have led to a remarkable increase in pacemaker sophistication, such that a wide range of different functions is now available. The most basic function of a pacemaker is to provide a 'safety net' for patients at risk of bradycardia. However, pacemakers that can terminate tachycardias and restore the synchronization of right and left ventricular contraction in heart failure are also available.

Pacemakers can either be **temporary**, to provide pacing in an emergency, or to tide patients over a short period of bradycardia (e.g. during a myocardial infarction) or until a permanent pacemaker can be implanted; or they can be **permanent**, in which case the battery, electronics and electrode(s) are all implanted within the patient. Temporary pacemakers are usually transvenous, but transoesophageal and transcutaneous pacing can also be used.

Patients seldom need pacing all the time, so both temporary and permanent pacemakers can be set up to monitor the heart's activity and provide impulses only when necessary. In the case of permanent pacemakers, this is an effective way of prolonging the lifetime of the battery, typically to between 7 and 15 years.

● Percussion pacing

Cardiac pacing can sometimes be achieved with no mechanical aids whatsoever. The technique of **percussion pacing** was first described in the 1960s and can help to maintain a good cardiac output in a bradycardic patient with considerably less trauma than chest compression. Percussion pacing is performed by delivering gentle blows to the praecordium (alongside the lower left sternal edge) to stimulate QRS complexes – the technique can be remarkably effective and can buy enough time to arrange further treatment as appropriate.

● Indications for temporary pacing

Patients awaiting permanent pacing

If a patient has a severely symptomatic bradycardia but permanent pacing cannot be undertaken within an acceptable time, temporary pacing may be used to support them in the interim.

Acute myocardial infarction

In acute **inferior** myocardial infarction, damage to the artery that supplies the atrioventricular (AV) node can cause complete heart block and bradycardia. Few patients need help with temporary pacing, as blood pressure is usually maintained despite the slow heart rate. Temporary pacing is needed in second-degree and third-degree AV block with symptoms or haemodynamic disturbance.

Acute **anterior** myocardial infarction often causes hypotension as a result of damage to the left ventricle. Extensive infarction may involve the bundle branches in the interventricular septum and cause bradycardia. Mortality is high. Temporary pacing and inotropic support are necessary for second-degree and third-degree AV block, even when the condition is asymptomatic.

Tachycardia

Some tachycardias (including AV re-entry tachycardia and ventricular tachycardia) can be terminated by **overdrive pacing**. This should only be undertaken under the guidance of someone experienced in the technique – contact a cardiologist for assistance.

Perioperative pacing

See page 229 for further information.

● Temporary pacemaker insertion and care

Once the decision to insert a temporary pacemaker has been made, you must ensure that:

- the pacing wire is inserted by a trained member of staff using aseptic technique
- X-ray screening time is kept to a minimum
- a 'breathable' dressing is applied to the wound

- a chest radiograph is requested (and looked at!) after the pacemaker has been inserted to check for pneumothorax
- the function of the pacemaker is monitored daily by checking the pacing threshold and ensuring the output is set at double the threshold
- the pacing wire does not dislodge
- the pacing wire is removed at the earliest opportunity to prevent infection
- the pacing wire is replaced, if still required, after 5 days, after which time the risk of infection increases sharply
- temporary pacing is not withheld in acute myocardial infarction because of thrombolysis (the external jugular, brachiocephalic or femoral veins can be used for intravenous access routes in these circumstances, as these are superficial and easily compressed to control bleeding).

Indications for permanent pacing

The decision to implant a *permanent* pacemaker must be made by a cardiologist, and you should seek their advice if you are uncertain about referring a patient. Generally speaking, the following are indications for a permanent pacemaker:

- **Third-degree AV block** with an episode of syncope or presyncope. Asymptomatic patients with acquired third-degree AV block and a ventricular rate less than 40 beats/min, or pauses greater than 3 s, should also be considered for pacing for prognostic reasons. Those with congenital third-degree AV block generally do not require pacing if they are asymptomatic, although they must be kept under regular review.
- **Second-degree AV block**, regardless of whether it is Mobitz type I or II, with an episode of symptomatic bradycardia.
- **Bifascicular** or **trifascicular block** with a clear history of syncope, or documented intermittent failure of the remaining fascicle.

- **Sick sinus syndrome** causing symptomatic bradycardia. Pacing is not usually necessary for patients with no symptoms.
- **Malignant vasovagal syndrome** is helped by pacing only if it is of the 'cardio-inhibitory' variety that causes a bradycardia.
- **Carotid sinus syndrome** is also only helped by pacing when it is of the cardio-inhibitory variety associated with a bradycardia.

● Selection of a permanent pacemaker

A wide choice of permanent pacemakers is now available, each offering a different pacing strategy. The cardiologist will be responsible for selecting the most appropriate type of unit to be inserted, as well as for providing long-term follow-up.

There is an internationally accepted code of up to five letters to describe the type of pacemaker. Each letter describes an aspect of the pacemaker's function (see Table 14.1).

Table 14.1 Pacemaker codes

Letter no.	Refers to	Code	Meaning
1	Chamber(s) paced	A	Atrium
		V	Ventricle
		D	Dual (both chambers)
2	Chamber(s) sensed	A	Atrium
		V	Ventricle
		D	Dual (both chambers)
		O	None
3	Response to sensing	I	Inhibition of pacemaker
		T	Triggering of pacemaker
		D	Inhibition or triggering
		O	None
4	Rate response	R	Rate-responsive pacemaker
5	Anti-tachycardia functions	P	Pacing of tachycardias
		S	Shock delivered
		D	Dual (pacing and shock)
		O	None

The following are some of the most commonly encountered pacemakers:

- **VVI**: this pacemaker has a single lead that senses activity in the ventricle. If no activity is detected, the pacemaker will take over control of the rhythm by pacing the ventricle via the same lead.
- **AAI**: this pacemaker also has a single lead, which is implanted in the atrium. It monitors atrial (P wave) activity. If normal atrial activity is not detected, it takes over by pacing the atria.
- **DDD**: this system has leads in both the atrium and the ventricle ('dual chamber'). It can both sense and pace via either lead. If it senses atrial activity but no ventricular activity, it will start pacing the ventricles in sequence with the atria. It can also pace the atria alone or, if AV conduction is blocked, pace the atria and ventricles sequentially.
- **AAIR, VVIR and DDDR**: the 'R' indicates that the pacemaker is rate responsive (see box below).

● Rate responsiveness

A rate-responsive pacemaker adjusts its pacing rate according to the patient's level of activity to mimic the physiological response to exercise. Several parameters can be monitored by pacemakers to determine the patient's level of activity, including vibration, respiration and blood temperature.

● Pacing and the ECG

Pacemakers activate depolarization with electrical impulses, and these appear as pacing 'spikes' on the ECG (Fig. 14.1). In ventricular pacing, a pacing spike will be followed by a broad QRS complex (because the depolarization is not conducted by the normal, fast-conduction pathways).

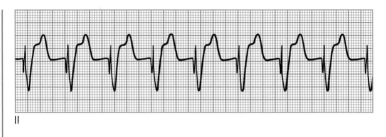

II

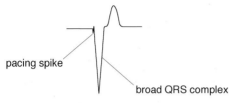

pacing spike

broad QRS complex

Fig. 14.1 Ventricular pacing

Key point:
- ventricular pacing spikes are followed by broad QRS complexes

When the atria are being paced via an atrial lead, the pacing spike will be followed by a P wave. This may be conducted normally via the AV junction and followed by a normal QRS complex. Alternatively, in dual-chamber sequential pacing, the P wave will be followed by a pacing spike from the ventricular lead and a broad QRS complex (Fig. 14.2).

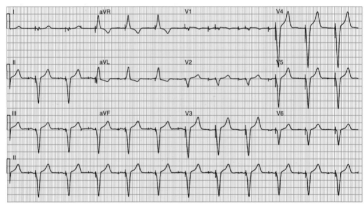

Fig. 14.2 Dual-chamber sequential pacing

Key points:
- atrial pacing spikes (small) are followed by P waves
- ventricular pacing spikes (large) are followed by broad QRS complexes

Failure of a pacing spike to be followed by depolarization indicates a problem with 'capture', and a cardiologist should be contacted to arrange a pacemaker check.

Pacemakers and surgery

Pacemakers are relevant in surgery for two reasons:

- permanent pacemakers and diathermy
- temporary prophylactic perioperative pacing.

Surgeons and anaesthetists must always be made aware if a patient undergoing surgery has a permanent pacemaker. Always ascertain the pacemaker type (patients usually carry an identification card with the pacemaker code on it) and the original indication for its insertion. It may also be advisable to arrange a check of the pacemaker before and after surgery.

Particular care must be taken during the operation to avoid interference with, or damage to, the pacemaker from diathermy. A particular risk of diathermy is that of inappropriate pacemaker inhibition, causing bradycardia or even asystole; it is therefore important to monitor the patient's ventricular rate closely throughout the procedure. To minimize the dangers, the 'active' diathermy electrode should be placed at least 15 cm from the pacemaker's generator box, and the 'indifferent' electrode as far from the box as possible.

Patients with certain cardiac conduction disorders who do *not* have a permanent pacemaker should be considered for a temporary pacemaker if they are about to undergo a procedure under general anaesthesia. Temporary pacing is indicated in:

- atrial fibrillation with a slow ventricular rate
- third-degree AV block
- second-degree AV block.

Pacing is not usually necessary for bifascicular block unless the patient has a history of presyncope or syncope. Consult a cardiologist for further guidance.

● Implantable cardioverter defibrillators

ICDs have proved to be invaluable in the management of life-threatening ventricular arrhythmias. Only a little larger than permanent pacemakers, they are implanted subcutaneously, usually in the same location as permanent pacemakers, although some of the older, bigger, units were implanted abdominally.

ICDs continually monitor the cardiac rhythm looking for ventricular arrhythmias. If an episode of ventricular tachycardia occurs, the device will normally begin by trying to overdrive pace the arrhythmia to terminate it. If that fails, the device will usually go on to deliver a shock. If ventricular fibrillation is detected, a shock is delivered as first-line treatment. The parameters by which ICDs diagnose arrhythmias and respond to them can be individually programmed into the device after it has been implanted, so that treatments most appropriate to the patient's condition can be chosen.

ICDs are expensive (costing around £20 000) but effective, and many trials having shown marked reduction in mortality. They are indicated for patients with a history of:

- ventricular fibrillation or ventricular tachycardia (not due to a transient or reversible cause)
- syncope (where haemodynamically significant ventricular arrhythmias can be induced during electrophysiological studies (EPS) and where drug treatment is ineffective or cannot be used)
- non-sustained ventricular tachycardia in the setting of ischaemic cardiomyopathy where ventricular arrhythmias can be induced during EPS and are not suppressible using Class I anti-arrhythmic agents.

ICDs are usually capable of acting as permanent pacemakers during episodes of bradycardia.

● Biventricular pacing: cardiac resynchronization treatment

In some patients with heart failure, the right and left ventricles do not contract simultaneously due to AV and intraventricular conduction delays. This can impair left ventricular contractility, making symptoms of heart failure worse.

Pacing both the right and the left ventricles can restore synchronization of right and left ventricular contraction, leading to improvements in quality of life and exercise tolerance, reduced mortality and reduced need for hospitalization in up to two-thirds of patients.

Cardiac resynchronization treatment is indicated in patients with advanced heart failure (New York Heart Association functional classes III and IV) with a left ventricular ejection fraction ≤35 per cent, who are in sinus rhythm with a QRS duration of ≥150 msec (or a QRS duration of 120–149 msec with confirmed mechanical dyssynchrony on echocardiography), and who are on optimal drug therapy. Further details can be found in Technology Appraisal TA120 from the National Institute for Health and Clinical Excellence (www.nice.org.uk).

Ambulatory ECG recording

The ECG is a key investigation in patients with palpitations. However, most patients who complain of palpitations only experience them intermittently. One of the limitations of the 12-lead ECG is that, in patients with a history of intermittent palpitations, the ECG is often entirely normal between episodes.

Although a 12-lead ECG recorded while the patient is asymptomatic might indicate the probable nature of the arrhythmia (for instance, the finding of a short PR interval makes atrioventricular re-entry tachycardia a likely diagnosis, whereas a long QT interval makes ventricular tachycardia (VT) more likely), there is no substitute for obtaining an ECG recording **during** an episode of palpitations. There are five ways in which this can be achieved:

- 24-h ambulatory ECG recording
- event recorder
- ECG 'on demand'
- bedside monitoring/telemetry (inpatient)
- implantable loop recorder.

Table 15.1 provides a guide to which modality of investigation is most likely to capture an ECG during an episode of palpitations, depending on the frequency of the patient's symptoms.

Table 15.1 Probability of capturing an episode of palpitations

Investigation method	Period between episodes		
	Days	Weeks	Months
24-h ambulatory ECG recording	+++	+	+
Event recorder	+++	++	+
ECG 'on demand'	+++*	+++*	+++*
Bedside monitoring/telemetry (inpatient)	+++	+	+
Implantable loop recorder	+++	+++	+++

+++, good; ++, fair; +, poor.
*Only helpful if the patient is able to obtain an ECG during a symptomatic episode.

● 24-h ambulatory ECG recording

The 24-h ambulatory ECG recording (Holter monitor) is one of the most frequently requested investigations in the assessment of patients with palpitations. The recorder is carried by the patient on a strap or belt and records the ECG via a small number of electrodes applied to the skin. The recording is usually made digitally onto a solid state memory card or, in older machines, onto a cassette tape. After the device is returned, the recording is analysed using appropriate software, looking for any rhythm disturbance.

One of the main drawbacks of the 24-h ambulatory ECG recorder is its short duration. Although recordings can take place over 48 h or even longer, the recording is usually only of value if the patient happens to experience an episode of palpitations while wearing it. If a patient's symptoms are occurring on a daily basis, or two or three times a week, there is a reasonable probability of capturing an ECG during a symptomatic episode. With less frequent symptoms, the 24-h ambulatory ECG recording is much less likely to be informative.

Patients with palpitations are often reassured that their 24-h ECG recording was normal and no further investigations are arranged. However, such reassurance cannot be given if the patient was asymptomatic during the recording. This kind of false reassurance is a cause of great concern, as even patients with life-threatening arrhythmias may well have entirely normal ECG recordings between events. The key question to ask any patient about their 24-h ECG recording is: 'Did you experience your typical symptoms during the recording?' If the answer is 'No', the recording should be regarded as non-diagnostic and further investigation may need to be arranged.

Patients should always keep a symptom diary during the recording to help their recollection of events, and should be asked to note the exact time that any events occurred. During analysis of the recording, particular attention must be paid to those periods of the recording during which symptoms occurred, to allow accurate correlation between the symptoms experienced by the patient and their cardiac rhythm at the time.

● Event recorder

Event recorders are usually carried by the patient for longer periods than 24-h or 48-h ambulatory ECG recorders, the main difference being that they are used only to record the ECG during symptomatic episodes rather than continuously. To use an event recorder, the patient must be able to activate the device whenever symptoms occur – a recording is then obtained for a predetermined duration (often around 30 s). With some devices, the patient can then transmit the recording back to the hospital by telephone for an immediate analysis of the cardiac rhythm.

There are two main types of event recorder: those that are continuously attached to the patient via ECG electrodes, and those that are only applied to the chest during an episode of palpitations. The former type is really just an extension of 24-h ambulatory ECG recording, the main difference being that the ECG is not recorded continuously, but instead is only recorded for a short period whenever the patient activates the device. Practical considerations (such as washing and skin irritation from the electrodes) mean that patients can usually only wear this type of event recorder for 7 days. The latter type is usually a small device that can be carried in the patient's pocket for as long as required. The device is held against the skin (usually over the anterior chest wall) and activated whenever symptoms occur.

Patients with relatively infrequent symptoms (occurring, for instance, on a weekly rather than a daily basis) can carry an event recorder in the hope of obtaining an ECG recording during a typical symptomatic episode. If the symptoms are less frequent (e.g. occurring every few months), an event recorder is unlikely to be helpful.

● ECG 'on demand'

In principle, one of the most effective ways to obtain an ECG recording during an episode of palpitations is to ask the patient to attend for an urgent ECG as soon as they notice the onset of symptoms. Practically, however, this approach poses a number of difficulties:

- The symptoms may not last long enough to give the patient time to reach a facility with an ECG machine.
- The patient may not have transport available and it may be inadvisable for them to drive or to travel unaccompanied while symptomatic.
- The patient may be asked to wait in line for an ECG when they arrive, by which time their symptoms may have resolved.

Nonetheless, this can be a rewarding approach, particularly if a patient's symptoms are relatively mild and infrequent (e.g. only occurring every few weeks or months) but last for long enough for them to reach a facility with an ECG machine. The patient should be given a form or letter (see the box below) and advised to take it to their nearest general practitioner or hospital accident and emergency department (or ECG department) when they develop symptoms. The letter should be on official notepaper and should request that whoever sees the patient must perform a 12-lead ECG **as soon as possible** if the patient presents with symptoms. The letter should also give an address to which a copy of the ECG should be sent **and**, in case the ECG goes astray, should ask that the patient also be given a copy to keep. The patient should then bring any ECGs recorded in this way to their next consultation.

● Suggested letter format for ECG 'on demand'
To Whom It May Concern

Re: [*insert patient's details here*]

The above-named patient is currently undergoing investigation for palpitations. He or she has been instructed to try to obtain a 12-lead ECG if he or she experiences a symptomatic episode.

If the patient presents to you with palpitations, please would you obtain a good-quality 12-lead ECG recording **as rapidly as possible** (before the symptoms resolve). Please note on the ECG recording whether the patient's symptoms were still present at the time of the recording.

I would be grateful if you would send a copy of the ECG to [*insert doctor's details here*]. Please also give a copy to the patient to bring to his or her next consultation.

Thank you.

[*Insert name and signature here*]

● Bedside monitoring/telemetry (inpatient)

If the palpitations are frequent (e.g. daily) and sufficiently troublesome to merit an urgent diagnosis, one option that is likely to yield a diagnosis is to admit the patient to hospital and use a bedside cardiac monitor (or telemetry). The patient should be instructed to inform the nursing staff immediately whenever he or she experiences palpitations so that the monitor can be checked and a recording obtained. Many bedside ECG monitors now incorporate diagnostic software that is sophisticated enough to detect most (but not all) significant arrhythmias, sound an alarm and store (or print out) a rhythm strip.

This approach can be effective at obtaining a diagnosis, but its limitations are that it can be expensive, it can be inconvenient for patients and it takes patients out of their 'everyday' environment and activities, which might affect the frequency of their symptoms.

● Implantable loop recorder

The patient who experiences severe but infrequent symptoms, such as unheralded syncope occurring once every few months, presents one of the most challenging problems. In this case the urgent need to identify a potentially dangerous rhythm disturbance (such as VT or intermittent third-degree atrioventricular block) is made more difficult by its infrequent occurrence. Even an event recorder is a rather hit-and-miss method of capturing symptomatic episodes and, if the patient loses consciousness, they may not be able to activate a recorder until after the rhythm disturbance has resolved and they have regained consciousness.

An implantable loop recorder (such as Medtronic's Reveal DX device) provides a useful means of attempting to capture an ECG during one of these infrequent episodes. The device is small (and has no attached leads) and is implanted subcutaneously in a similar position to a permanent pacemaker. It contains a battery (which lasts approximately 14 months) and a digital recorder that monitors the ECG and records a rhythm strip. The recorder works on a loop principle, so that the earliest rhythm recording is continuously overwritten by the latest on a continuous 'rolling' basis. At any one time around 20 min of the current cardiac rhythm are stored in the device's memory, although the amount of storage available varies according to the device and its settings.

If an event occurs, the recording loop can be 'frozen' by the patient using an activation device that is held against the recorder – this recording can then be downloaded at a later date by the centre where the unit was implanted. The latest devices also contain diagnostic software that can be programmed to identify and store asymptomatic rhythm disturbances. There is sufficient memory in the device to record several loops before a download is necessary.

The implantable loop recorder represents a useful way to record the ECG in those patients whose symptoms are infrequent but nonetheless worrying. Its usefulness has to be weighed against the need for an invasive procedure (with the associated risks of scarring and infection) and the cost of the device, although the cost is somewhat offset by the reduced need for multiple non-invasive ambulatory recordings.

16 Exercise ECG testing

The exercise ECG can be a valuable tool for the assessment of patients with ischaemic heart disease and exercise-related arrhythmias. However, failure to interpret exercise ECGs correctly limits their usefulness.

In this chapter, we will help you to answer the following questions:

- What are the indications for an exercise ECG?
- What are the risks of an exercise ECG?
- How do I perform an exercise ECG?
- When do I stop an exercise ECG?
- How do I interpret an exercise ECG?

● What are the indications for an exercise ECG?

Exercise ECG testing can be useful in:

- diagnosing chest pain
- risk stratification in stable angina
- risk stratification after myocardial infarction
- assessing exercise-induced arrhythmias
- assessing the need for a permanent pacemaker
- assessing exercise tolerance
- assessing response to treatment.

Exercise ECG testing should always be undertaken with a specific question in mind, and an appreciation of its limitations. In particular, it should only be performed if the information you are likely to gain outweighs the potential (albeit small) risks.

● What are the risks of an exercise ECG?

As with all procedures, exercise ECG testing carries risks:

- morbidity of 2.4 in 10 000
- mortality of 1 in 10 000 (within 1 week of testing).

To minimize the risks, always take a patient history and perform an examination to check for **absolute** contraindications to exercise ECG testing (Table 16.1).

Table 16.1 Absolute contraindications to an exercise ECG

- Recent myocardial infarction (within 7 days)
- Unstable angina (rest pain within previous 48 h)
- Severe aortic stenosis or hypertrophic obstructive cardiomyopathy
- Acute myocarditis
- Acute pericarditis
- Uncontrolled hypertension
  - systolic BP >250 mmHg
  - diastolic BP >120 mmHg
- Uncontrolled heart failure
- Recent thromboembolic episode (pulmonary or systemic)
- Acute febrile illness

In addition, there are several **relative** contraindications to exercise testing, in the presence of which the test should only be performed with a full awareness of the increased risks involved and under close medical supervision (Table 16.2).

● How do I perform an exercise ECG?

Unless the exercise test is being performed to assess the effectiveness of treatment, patients should be advised to tail-off

Table 16.2 Relative contraindications to an exercise ECG

- Recent myocardial infarction (within 7 days to 1 month)*
- Known severe coronary artery disease
- Known serious risk of arrhythmia
- Mild or moderate aortic stenosis or hypertrophic obstructive cardiomyopathy
- Pulmonary hypertension
- Significant left ventricular dysfunction
- Aneurysm (ventricular or aortic)
- Highly abnormal resting ECG†
  - left or right bundle branch block
  - digoxin effect
- Frail patients

*A submaximal exercise test should be used.
†A myocardial perfusion scan can be considered instead.

any existing anti-anginal treatment over the 3 days before the test. They can use sublingual glyceryl trinitrate until 1 h before the test.

On the day of the test, ensure that two people trained in cardiopulmonary resuscitation (CPR) are present for supervision and that all the necessary drugs and equipment for CPR are available.

After explaining the test to the patient and checking for contraindications (see previous section), decide which exercise protocol to use. There are many different protocols, but the two most commonly used are:

- the Bruce protocol
- the modified Bruce protocol.

The modified Bruce protocol begins with a lighter workload than the Bruce protocol, and is particularly suitable for frail patients or those being assessed after a recent myocardial infarction (Fig. 16.1).

After reviewing the patient's resting ECG and checking their blood pressure, they can commence exercise. Monitor their symptoms and ECG throughout, and check their blood pressure every 3 min. Reasons for stopping the test are discussed below.

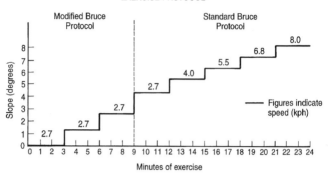

Fig. 16.1 The Bruce and modified Bruce protocols

After the completion of exercise, continue to monitor the patient's ECG and blood pressure until any symptoms or ECG changes have fully resolved.

● What is a MET?

The workload at each level of an exercise protocol can be expressed in terms of metabolic equivalents (or METs). One MET, the rate of oxygen consumption by a normal person at rest, is 3.5 mL/kg per min. To perform the activities of daily living requires 5 METs.

● When do I stop an exercise ECG?

One indicator of a good prognosis is the ability to achieve a target heart rate with no symptoms or major ECG changes. The target heart rate is calculated as follows:

Target heart rate = 220 minus patient's age (in years)

However, several events may require the exercise test to be stopped before the target heart rate is reached. The test *must* be stopped if:

- the patient asks for the test to be stopped
- the systolic blood pressure falls by >20 mmHg
- the heart rate falls by >10 beats/min
- sustained ventricular or supraventricular arrhythmias occur.

In addition, you should consider stopping the test if the patient develops:

- >2 mm ST segment depression and chest pain
- >3 mm asymptomatic ST segment depression
- conduction disturbance and chest pain
- non-sustained ventricular tachycardia
- dizziness
- marked or disproportionate breathlessness
- severe fatigue or exhaustion.

● How do I interpret an exercise ECG?

If the exercise ECG was done to induce an exercise-related arrhythmia, it should be fairly clear whether the test has succeeded in doing so. The interpretation of arrhythmias is the subject of the earlier chapters in this book. Repeating the exercise test once the patient has been established on treatment can be helpful in assessing its efficacy.

Exercise ECGs performed for ischaemic heart disease are often poorly interpreted, and part of the reason for this is a failure to appreciate their limitations. Exercise ECG testing is *not* a 'gold standard' test for ischaemic heart disease – the sensitivity of an exercise test is 45–68 per cent and specificity 75–90 per cent and so you should be careful about reporting tests in 'black or white' terms such as 'positive' or 'negative'. It may be more useful instead to estimate the probability that a patient has coronary artery disease (see below).

The most common indicator of coronary artery disease on exercise is the development of ST segment depression, and the greater the depression, the higher the probability of coronary artery disease. However, care must be taken when measuring ST segment depression during exercise, as depression of the **J point** (the junction of the S wave and ST segment) is normal. The ST segment slopes upwards sharply after the J point, and returns to the baseline within 60 ms (1.5 small squares). You must therefore measure ST segment depression **80 ms (2 small squares) beyond the J point** (Fig. 16.2).

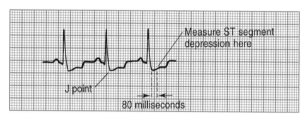

Fig. 16.2 The J point

Key points:
- the J point is the junction of the S wave and ST segment
- measure ST segment depression 80 ms after the J point

ST segment depression is not the only noteworthy result, however. T wave inversion may develop during exercise, as may bundle branch block, although these can occur without major coronary artery disease. A fall in systolic blood pressure often indicates severe coronary artery disease.

The ECGs in Fig. 16.3 were recorded in a patient with three-vessel coronary artery disease, and show the ST segment changes before, during and after exercise.

The probability of a patient having coronary artery disease depends on:

- gender – the prevalence of coronary disease is greater in men, so a positive test is more likely to be a true positive in

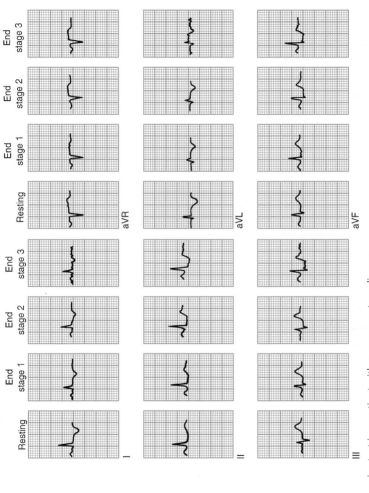

Fig. 16.3 Exercise test in a patient with coronary artery disease

Key point: ● inferolateral ST segment depression during exercise

(Continued)

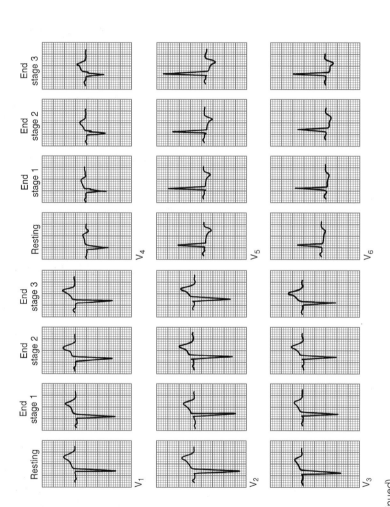

Fig. 16.3 (Continued)

Table 16.3 Probability (per cent) of coronary artery disease according to age, sex and exercise test findings

Age (years)	ST segment depression (mm)	Symptoms Men				Women			
		None	Non-anginal chest pain	Atypical angina	Typical angina	None	Non-anginal chest pain	Atypical angina	Typical angina
30–39	0–0.5	<1	1	6	25	<1	<1	1	7
	0.5–1.0	2	5	21	68	<1	1	4	24
	1.0–1.5	4	10	38	83	1	2	9	42
	1.5–2.0	8	19	55	91	1	3	16	59
	2.0–2.5	18	38	76	96	3	8	33	79
	>2.5	43	68	92	99	11	24	63	93
40–49	0–0.5	1	4	16	61	<1	1	3	22
	0.5–1.0	5	13	44	86	1	3	12	53
	1.0–1.5	11	26	64	94	2	6	25	72
	1.5–2.0	20	41	78	97	4	11	39	84
	2.0–2.5	39	65	91	99	10	24	63	93
	>2.5	69	87	97	>99	28	53	86	98
50–59	0–0.5	2	6	25	73	1	2	10	47
	0.5–1.0	9	20	57	91	3	8	31	78
	1.0–1.5	19	37	75	96	7	16	50	89
	1.5–2.0	31	53	86	98	12	28	67	94
	2.0–2.5	54	75	94	99	27	50	84	98
	>2.5	81	91	98	>99	56	78	95	99
60–69	0–0.5	3	8	32	79	2	5	21	69
	0.5–1.0	11	26	65	94	7	17	52	90
	1.0–1.5	23	45	81	97	15	33	72	95
	1.5–2.0	37	62	90	99	25	49	83	98
	2.0–2.5	61	81	96	>99	47	72	93	99
	>2.5	85	94	99	>99	76	90	98	>99

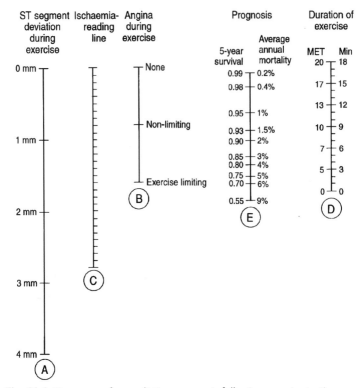

Fig. 16.4 Nomogram for predicting prognosis following exercise testing (Adapted from Mark DB, Shaw L, Harrell FE Jr, *et al*. *N Engl J Med* 1991;**325**:849–53. Copyright 1996, Massachusetts Medical Society. All rights reserved.)

How to use:
- Mark on line A the maximum ST segment deviation seen during exercise
- Mark on line B the degree of angina during exercise
- Join the marks on lines A and B with a straight line
- Mark the point where this line crosses line C (the 'ischaemia-reading line')
- Mark on line D the duration of exercise (Bruce protocol) or METS achieved
- Join the marks on lines C and D with a straight line
- Where this line crosses line E, read off the patient's predicted mortality

a man but more likely to be a false positive result in a woman
- age – the prevalence of coronary disease increases with advancing age, so a positive result is more likely to be a true positive in an older person but a false positive in a younger person
- ST segment depression – the greater the degree of ST segment depression, the earlier ST segment depression appears and the more leads affected, the greater the probability of coronary disease
- accompanying symptoms – typical symptoms of angina accompanied by ST segment depression increases the probability of coronary disease.

Table 16.3 allows you to estimate a patient's probability of coronary artery disease based on these parameters. The results of exercise ECG testing also allow for risk stratification by using a nomogram, such as the one in Figure 16.4, to predict mortality.

Cardiopulmonary resuscitation

Many cardiac arrests are poorly managed because of disorganization of the cardiac arrest team and a lack of knowledge about recommended procedures by its members. In particular, arrhythmias are frequently incorrectly diagnosed and treated. The rapid identification and treatment of arrhythmias are a cornerstone of successful cardiopulmonary resuscitation (CPR), and for this reason we have included this section on CPR to help you answer the following questions:

- How do I perform adult basic life support outside hospital?
- How do I perform inhospital resuscitation?
- How do I perform advanced life support?
  - Shockable rhythms
  - Non-shockable rhythms
- How do I diagnose the arrhythmias?
- How should I use the defibrillator?
- How do I manage peri-arrest arrhythmias?
  - Bradycardia
  - Tachycardia
- How should I direct others during the arrest?
- What should I do after the arrest?

This chapter is based on the Resuscitation Council (UK) Guidelines 2005. If you would like to learn more about advanced life support, there is no substitute for attending a formal training course. In the UK such courses are coordinated by the

Resuscitation Council (UK) and contact details can be found in the 'Further reading' section at the end of this book.

Current teaching in CPR emphasizes the chain of survival – four interventions that contribute to a successful outcome. These are:

- early access to help (from emergency services or a cardiac arrest team)
- early basic life support (BLS) to buy time
- early defibrillation (where appropriate)
- early advanced life support to stabilize the patient.

All four links in the chain must be strong to maximize the chances of a successful outcome. All four elements of the chain of survival are covered in this chapter.

● How do I perform adult basic life support outside hospital?

The concept of BLS assumes that no special equipment is initially available, as might be the case if someone collapses in the street. This section assumes that BLS is taking place outside the hospital environment and that only a single rescuer is present. Inhospital resuscitation will be covered in the next section.

The current resuscitation guidelines have simplified BLS to aid the learning and retention of BLS skills, and have also increased the number of chest compressions compared with earlier guidelines.

If you witness someone collapse, or find someone apparently unresponsive, first of all ensure that you and everyone around you (including the victim) is safe. Next, assess whether the victim is responsive by gently shaking him by the shoulders and asking loudly, 'Are you all right?'. If the victim responds, try not to move him (unless he is in danger) and try to ascertain what is wrong. Get help if needed, and reassess the victim regularly.

If the victim does not respond, shout for help. Turn the victim onto his back and open his airway with a head-tilt and chin-lift manoeuvre. Look, listen and feel for normal breathing for no more than 10 s – if in doubt, it is better to assume that the victim's breathing is *not* normal.

If the victim is breathing normally, turn him into the recovery position and get help (even if you have to leave the patient). Then check regularly to ensure that normal breathing continues.

If the victim is not breathing normally, ask someone to call an ambulance (or do this yourself, even if you have to leave the victim). Then commence chest compressions at a rate of 100 compressions/min, depressing the sternum by 4–5 cm with each compression.

After 30 chest compressions, open the airway again (head-tilt, chin-lift) and, while pinching the victim's nose, give two effective rescue breaths. Then continue with chest compressions, alternating between 30 chest compressions and 2 rescue breaths (30:2 ratio). Only stop to recheck the victim if he starts breathing normally – otherwise, continue the BLS uninterrupted.

If there is more than one rescuer, swap places (with minimal interruption to BLS) every min.

If you are unwilling or unable to give rescue breaths, give chest compressions continuously at a rate of 100/min, stopping to recheck the victim only if he starts breathing normally.

Continue resuscitation until qualified help arrives, the patient starts breathing normally or you become exhausted.

● How do I perform inhospital resuscitation?

The BLS technique described above is most useful in the community setting where just one rescuer is present. Things are somewhat different in the hospital setting and the distinction between basic and advanced life support is more blurred. The latest guidelines take this into account and include a new section on inhospital resuscitation.

When a patient 'collapses' in hospital, first of all ensure your own safety and the safety of those around you. Shout for help immediately, and then assess the patient for responsiveness as described above.

If the patient is responsive, request urgent medical help and, while awaiting this, assess the patient using the ABCDE (Airway – Breathing – Circulation – Disability and neurological Damage – Exposure) approach. The patient should be given oxygen, ECG monitoring electrodes should be attached and venous access obtained.

If the patient is unresponsive, ensure help is on its way and then turn the patient onto his back and open his airway (checking for any obstruction, and taking appropriate care with regard to any possible cervical spine injury). Look, listen and feel for normal breathing for no more than 10 s, taking care not to mistake agonal breaths for normal breathing. If you are experienced in doing so, you can also check for a carotid pulse during or immediately after the breathing check. If a pulse or other signs of life are present, proceed as per the responsive patient above.

If there is no pulse or other signs of life, one person should commence CPR while the others call the resuscitation team and fetch the resuscitation trolley – if you are the only person present, you should leave the patient and summon help before continuing. Give 30 chest compressions at a rate of 100 compressions/min, depressing the sternum by 4–5 cm with each compression.

The patient's airway should be maintained and ventilation given using the equipment available (which may include a pocket mask, oral airway or laryngeal mask airway). Use supplemental oxygen as soon as it is available. If a trained and experienced staff member is able to perform tracheal intubation they should do so. Once the airway is secure, chest compressions should continue at 100/min and lung ventilations at 10/min.

Once a defibrillator is available, attach the electrodes to the patient and assess the rhythm, attempting defibrillation where appropriate (see below). Chest compressions should be restarted immediately after the defibrillation attempt without pausing to assess the pulse or rhythm. Resuscitation should continue until the resuscitation team arrives or until the patient shows signs of life.

In cases where the patient has a pulse but is not breathing (respiratory arrest), ventilation should be performed at 10 breaths/min and the pulse should be rechecked every minute. This should only be done by someone experienced in assessing the carotid pulse – if the presence of a pulse is uncertain, commence chest compression.

● Assessing the carotid pulse

Assessment of the carotid pulse no longer forms part of the standard protocol unless the rescuer is skilled in doing it. This is because assessment of the carotid pulse is time consuming and the decision about the presence or absence of the pulse is, in unskilled hands, often wrong. The carotid pulse should only be assessed by those experienced in doing so. If there is uncertainty about the presence of a carotid pulse, chest compression should be performed.

Where a patient has a witnessed and monitored cardiac arrest, and a defibrillator is not immediately available, you can consider giving a single precordial thump (if you have been trained in the technique) after calling for help.

How do I perform advanced life support?

Cardiac arrest arrhythmias are divided into 'shockable' rhythms (ventricular fibrillation (VF)/pulseless ventricular tachycardia (VT)) and 'non-shockable' rhythms (pulseless electrical activity (PEA) and asystole). The key difference is the need for defibrillation in the shockable group. Other aspects of managing the patient are common to the two groups. Advanced life support is summarized in the algorithm in Figure 17.1.

Shockable rhythms (VF/pulseless VT)

Where a shockable rhythm is present, one shock (150–360 J biphasic or 360 J monophasic) should be given followed by immediate resumption of CPR (as described in the earlier sections) for 2 min.

After the 2 min have elapsed, pause briefly to reassess the cardiac rhythm and, if VF/pulseless VT persists, give a second shock (150–360 J biphasic or 360 J monophasic). Immediately resume CPR for another 2 min.

After the 2 min have elapsed, pause briefly to reassess the cardiac rhythm and, if VF/pulseless VT persists, administer adrenaline 1 mg intravenously (IV) followed by a third shock (150–360 J biphasic or 360 J monophasic). Immediately resume CPR for another 2 min.

After the 2 min have elapsed, pause briefly to reassess the cardiac rhythm and, if VF/pulseless VT persists, administer amiodarone 300 mg IV followed by a fourth shock (150–360 J biphasic or 360 J monophasic). Immediately resume CPR for another 2 min.

Adrenaline 1 mg IV should be given immediately before alternate shocks (i.e. every 3–5 min) and, if VF/pulseless VT persists, a shock should be given after every 2-min period of CPR. If organized electrical activity occurs at any point, check for a

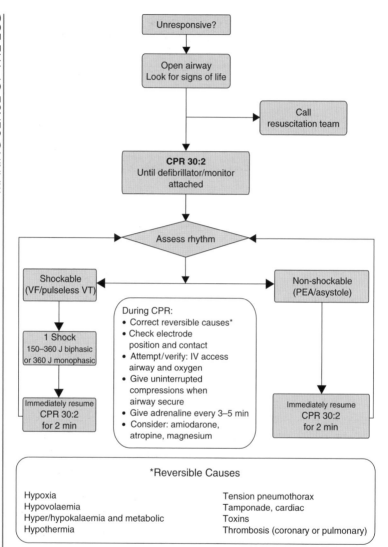

Fig. 17.1 Adult advanced life support algorithm

Source: Resuscitation Guidelines 2005. Reproduced with the kind permission of the Resuscitation Council (UK). IV, intravenous.

pulse. If a pulse is present, start post-resuscitation care. If a pulse is absent despite organized electrical activity, switch to the non-shockable arm of the algorithm (see Fig. 17.1). Similarly, if asystole is seen, switch to the non-shockable arm of the algorithm.

Non-shockable rhythms (PEA and asystole)

Where a non-shockable rhythm is present, it is particularly important to look for an underlying treatable cause for the arrest (Table 17.1). Successful resuscitation is unlikely unless a treatable cause is present.

Table 17.1 Potentially reversible causes of cardiac arrest

- Hypoxia
- Hypovolaemia
- Hyperkalaemia, hypokalaemia, hypocalcaemia, acidaemia, and other metabolic disorders
- Hypothermia
- Tension pneumothorax
- Tamponade
- Toxic substances
- Thromboembolism (pulmonary embolus/coronary thrombosis)

Pulseless electrical activity

Once PEA has been identified, commence CPR (at a ratio of 30:2) and give adrenaline 1 mg IV as soon as intravenous access is available. Once the airway has been secured, chest compressions can then continue without interruption for ventilation.

After 2 min have elapsed, pause briefly to reassess the cardiac rhythm and, if there is no change in the ECG, immediately resume CPR. This loop can be repeated for as long as is appropriate. Administer adrenaline 1 mg IV every second loop (i.e. every 3–5 min).

If the ECG changes and there is organized electrical activity, check for a pulse and, if present, start post-resuscitation care (see below). If no pulse is present, return to the loops of CPR as described above.

Asystole and slow pulseless electrical activity

Once asystole or slow PEA (ventricular rate <60 beats per minute) has been identified, commence CPR (at a ratio of 30:2) and check that the ECG electrodes are correctly connected (without interrupting CPR). Give adrenaline 1 mg IV and atropine 3 mg IV (once only) as soon as intravenous access is available. Once the airway has been secured, chest compressions can then continue without interruption for ventilation.

After 2 min have elapsed, pause briefly to reassess the cardiac rhythm and, if there is no change in the ECG, immediately resume CPR. This loop can be repeated for as long as is appropriate. Administer adrenaline 1 mg IV every second loop (i.e. every 3–5 min).

If VF/pulseless VT occurs at any point, switch to the shockable rhythm algorithm.

● How do I diagnose the arrhythmias?

Remember: time is of the essence. Rapid and correct identification and treatment of cardiac rhythm abnormalities are central to the delivery of effective advanced life support.

You must be able to recognize with confidence each of the four arrhythmias that occur in cardiac arrest:

- VF
- pulseless VT
- asystole
- PEA.

In addition, you should know how to manage three arrhythmias (discussed later in this chapter) that may appear during or shortly after cardiac arrest:

- bradycardia
- narrow-complex tachycardia
- broad-complex tachycardia.

Ventricular fibrillation

Ventricular fibrillation is the commonest initial arrhythmia causing cardiac arrest and appears as a chaotic rhythm on the ECG (Fig. 17.2). If the monitor is faulty, or the gain turned too low, it can be mistaken for asystole.

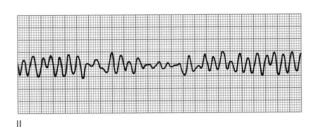

II

Fig. 17.2 Ventricular fibrillation

Key point: • chaotic ventricular activity

Pulseless ventricular tachycardia

Pulseless ventricular tachycardia appears as a broad-complex rapid cardiac rhythm (Fig. 17.3), and can cause haemodynamic collapse (hence 'pulseless').

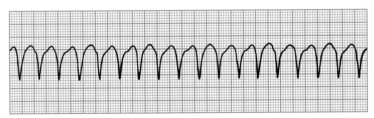

II

Fig. 17.3 Ventricular tachycardia

Key point: • broad-complex tachycardia

Asystole

Asystole implies there is no spontaneous electrical cardiac activity, and thus the ECG shows no QRS complexes (Fig. 17.4). P waves may persist for a short time after the onset of ventricular asystole (and are an indicator that the patient may respond to ventricular pacing). Beware of diagnosing asystole when you see a completely flat line on the monitor – there is usually some baseline drift in asystole and the line is seldom completely flat. A perfectly flat line is more likely to be due to a faulty electrode or connection.

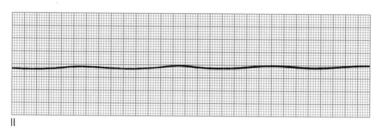

II

Fig. 17.4 Asystole

Key point: • no spontaneous electrical activity

Pulseless electrical activity

Pulseless electrical activity is sometimes called electromechanical dissociation, and occurs when the heart continues to work electrically (the ECG continues to show QRS complexes, Fig. 17.5), but fails to provide a circulation. Reasons for this include massive pulmonary embolism (obstructing blood flow), large myocardial infarction (causing mechanical 'weakness' of the heart muscle) and severe haemorrhage (loss of circulating volume).

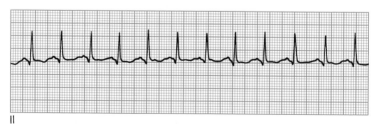

II

Fig. 17.5 Pulseless electrical activity

Key point: • QRS complexes (in the absence of a cardiac output)

> ● Cardiac rhythms in PEA
>
> It is important to remember that PEA can exist in conjunction with *any* of the cardiac rhythms that would normally sustain a circulation, not just sinus rhythm. Patients with atrial fibrillation or with an atrioventricular (AV) re-entry tachycardia, for instance, should normally have a pulse – in the absence of a pulse, they have PEA.

Having confidently diagnosed the rhythm disorder, move on quickly to provide the appropriate treatment.

● How should I use the defibrillator?

Defibrillation is used during a cardiac arrest to convert the heart from an abnormal rhythm to sinus rhythm (or, at least, to a rhythm that restores a cardiac output). Hence, you must use the defibrillator when you have diagnosed:

- VF
- pulseless VT.

> ● 'Fine' VF
>
> In previous versions of the advanced life support guidelines, it was recommended that defibrillation should be attempted where there was uncertainty about whether the patient was in asystole or in 'fine' VF. Current guidance has reversed this advice. It is now thought that if 'fine' VF is present, good quality CPR will improve the amplitude of the ECG waveform (making the diagnosis of VF clearer) and also enhance the chance of successful defibrillation.

There is no point in defibrillating a patient if they are in asystole. Defibrillation just changes one rhythm to another – it will not restart the heart when there is no initial rhythm. There is also no point in defibrillating pulseless electrical activity. By definition, the heart is working normally electrically – you have to find a mechanical reason for the lack of a cardiac output.

Ensure you are familiar with the defibrillators used in your workplace, as you cannot afford to waste time should you need to use one. Many units now use biphasic (rather than monophasic) defibrillators – these lower the defibrillation threshold and so lower shock energies (150–360 J) may be required compared to the higher shock energy of a monophasic device (360 J).

Apply electrode jelly or preferably gel pads to the skin below the paddles, but do not spread jelly between the paddles as this can cause a 'short circuit'. Note also that some gel pads need replacing between shocks.

After warning everyone to stand clear, perform a 'visual sweep' to check that:

- everyone (including yourself!) is clear of the patient and the bed
- no-one is touching drip stands connected to the patient
- any oxygen mask/nasal cannulae are at least 1 m away from the patient's chest
- all transdermal medication patches have been removed from the patient (risk of burns if they have a metal backing)
- the paddles are at least 15 cm from any permanent pacemaker or implantable cardioverter defibrillator box.

Finally, look one last time at the monitor to check the rhythm has not changed and, if appropriate, proceed to deliver the direct current (DC) shocks (as described in the appropriate protocol) without delay.

● How do I manage peri-arrest arrhythmias?

You must be able to recognize and be prepared to treat promptly any arrhythmia that develops during or shortly after cardiac arrest. Always be alert to adverse signs that will help determine the response to the arrhythmia (Table 17.2).

Table 17.2 Adverse clinical signs during arrhythmias

- Systolic blood pressure <90 mmHg
- Low cardiac output (poor perfusion, impaired conscious level)
- Excessive tachycardia (>200/min for narrow-complex tachycardia, >150/min for broad-complex tachycardia)
- Excessive bradycardia (<40/min)
- Heart failure (pulmonary or peripheral congestion)
- Myocardial ischaemia (chest pain or ST segment changes)

Bradycardia

You should quickly assess the patient's ECG and clinical condition, as these will help you decide the likelihood of their condition deteriorating. A ventricular rate <40/min is regarded as excessively slow, although patients may be acutely unwell even at higher rates if they have poor underlying cardiac function. The presence of adverse clinical signs is an indication for atropine 500 mcg IV.

If the response to atropine is unsatisfactory, or if there is a risk of asystole (Table 17.3), you should seek expert help with regard to transvenous pacing. In the meantime, you can give more doses of atropine (up to a maximum of 3 mg) and/or an infusion of adrenaline 2–10 mcg/min. Other drugs that can be useful in increasing the heart rate include aminophylline, isoprenaline and dopamine. You can also consider the use of transcutaneous pacing which can be very effective as a short-term measure, although it can be uncomfortable for the patient.

Table 17.3 Predictors of asystole

- Recent asystole
- Mobitz type II AV block
- Third-degree AV block with broad QRS complexes
- Ventricular pause >3 s

SEEK HELP

Expert help may be needed for patients with a peri-arrest bradycardia where there is a risk of asystole or which does not respond to atropine.

Tachycardia

A tachycardic patient with adverse clinical signs (see Table 17.2, p. 263) should be considered for urgent cardioversion with synchronized direct current (DC) shock (up to three attempts) under sedation or general anaesthesia. A loading dose of amiodarone 300 mg IV (given over 10–20 min) can be given if cardioversion fails to restore sinus rhythm, and cardioversion can then be reattempted once the loading dose has been administered. The loading dose can be followed by an infusion of another 900 mg IV over the next 24 h.

If the patient is stable, then the next step is to determine whether their tachycardia is narrow complex (QRS complex width <0.12 s) or broad complex.

Narrow-complex tachycardias

Irregular narrow-complex tachycardia is usually atrial fibrillation, or it may be atrial flutter with variable AV block. This can be rate-controlled with an intravenous beta blocker or intravenous digoxin (or, if of recent onset, the use of intravenous amiodarone may be effective in chemically cardioverting the patient to sinus rhythm).

Regular narrow-complex tachycardia may be due to:

- sinus tachycardia
- AVRT/AVNRT
- atrial flutter with regular AV block.

Vagal manoeuvres such as the Valsalva manoeuvre or carotid sinus massage may either cardiovert the arrhythmia (in the case of AVRT/AVNRT) or slow it down, making identification of atrial activity easier (in the case of sinus tachycardia and atrial flutter). Adenosine can also be used to block the AV node, with an initial dose of 6 mg IV (as a rapid bolus), followed if necessary with up to two more boluses of 12 mg IV.

Broad-complex tachycardias

Regular broad-complex tachycardia will be due either to VT or to a supraventricular tachycardia (SVT) with aberrant conduction. An SVT with bundle branch block can be treated in the same way as a regular narrow-complex tachycardia (see above). VT, or any rhythm where there is uncertainty about whether it is VT or not, can be treated in a stable patient with an infusion of amiodarone 300 mg IV (over 20–60 min) followed by 900 mg over 24 h.

Irregular broad-complex tachycardia may be due to:

- atrial fibrillation with aberrant conduction (which should be treated as for irregular narrow-complex tachycardia – see above)
- atrial fibrillation with pre-excitation (for which you should seek urgent expert help)
- polymorphic VT, which should be treated by stopping any pro-arrhythmic drugs and correcting any electrolyte abnormalities, and by giving magnesium sulphate 2 g IV over 10 min. Seek expert help as this is a hazardous arrhythmia. Urgent cardioversion may be needed if the patient becomes unstable.

● How should I direct others during the arrest?

A poorly trained and inexperienced arrest team will conduct a cardiac arrest in a disorganized manner. It is essential that all members of the team are familiar with basic and advanced life support guidelines and that the most experienced person present takes overall control of the situation.

While diagnosing the arrhythmias and taking decisions accordingly, the team leader must direct others by giving clear instructions to specified individuals. Ideally, there should be one member of the team for each of the following tasks:

- chest compression (swapping with others at 2-min intervals)
- defibrillation
- ventilating and/or intubating the patient
- obtaining intravenous access
- drawing up the necessary drugs
- keeping a record of events, and counting the seconds out loud whenever CPR is interrupted.

The team leader should also discuss with the rest of the team when further resuscitation appears futile and, if the others are in agreement, terminate resuscitation efforts.

● What should I do after the arrest?

After the return of a spontaneous circulation (ROSC), the patient will need observation and monitoring, ideally on an intensive or coronary care unit. Particularly important is the management of the patient's airway and breathing, especially if their conscious level is reduced, and artificial ventilation may be needed.

You will need to monitor:

- airway and breathing (including pulse oximetry)
- vital signs (pulse, blood pressure (preferably via an arterial line) and temperature)

- peripheral perfusion
- cardiac rhythm
- neurological status (including Glasgow Coma Score)
- urine output and fluid balance.

In addition you need to check:

- arterial blood gases
- blood urea and electrolytes (including K^+, Mg^{2+} and Ca^{2+})
- chest radiograph
- blood glucose
- 12-lead ECG
- full blood count.

These post-arrest investigations can be remembered by the mnemonic ABCDEF (**A**rterial blood gases; **B**iochemistry – blood urea and electrolytes; **C**hest X-ray; **D**extrose – blood glucose; **E**CG – 12-lead ECG; **F**ull blood count).

Finally, do not forget the patient's relatives. Speak to them as soon as possible after the arrest.

A history of ⓲ the ECG

The development of the ECG as a clinically useful tool began in the latter half of the nineteenth century and rapidly developed in the early twentieth century, such that by the 1940s the standard 12-lead ECG had taken on the appearance that is still recognizable today. In this chapter we chart the history of the ECG from the earliest experiments up to the present day.

● The electrical basis of the heartbeat

During the nineteenth century there was much interest in the role of electrical activity in the body, and the electrical basis of skeletal muscle contraction became well recognized. It was simple to show that the gastrocnemius muscle of a frog would contract if the attached sciatic nerve were stimulated electrically. In 1856, two German experimenters, Rudolph von Köllicker and Heinrich Müller, accidentally allowed the sciatic nerve from one frog to come into contact with an exposed beating heart from another. They noticed that the gastrocnemius muscle attached to the sciatic nerve began to twitch in time with the contractions of the exposed heart, demonstrating for the first time that the generation of the heartbeat also had an electrical basis.

● Development of recording devices

The next step in the development of the ECG was the invention of a device that would record the heart's electrical activity.

A variety of devices were developed in the nineteenth century that allowed variations in small electrical currents to be measured, all of which consisted (in one way or another) of devices that would move as the current varied, and that movement could then by recorded on a suitable strip of paper. A device called a Thompson siphon recorder was used by the electrical engineer Alexander Muirhead, working at St Bartholomew's Hospital in London, to record the first human ECG around 1870.

The Thompson siphon recorder was superseded by the capillary electrometer, invented by Gabriel Lippmann in the early 1870s. In this device, a column of mercury was placed in electrical contact with the body and variations in electrical current would cause expansion or contraction of the mercury column. These changes in the mercury column were magnified and projected onto photographic paper, allowing the changes to be recorded.

By 1876 Étienne-Jules Marey was using Lippmann's capillary electrometer to obtain ECG recordings from an exposed frog's heart, and by 1878 two British physiologists, John Burdon Sanderson and Fredrick Page, had shown that recordings of the frog heart's electrical activity consisted of two phases. These phases later became known as the QRS complex and the T wave.

Although Alexander Muirhead may have been the first to record a human ECG, the first to publish a human ECG (in 1887) was Augustus D Waller. While working at St Mary's Hospital, London, Waller used a capillary electrometer to record the ECG of a laboratory technician, Thomas Goswell.

● Einthoven and the string galvanometer

The Dutch physiologist Willem Einthoven, who witnessed a demonstration by Waller at the First International Congress of Physiology in Switzerland in 1889, went on to refine the technique of ECG recording. Einthoven worked hard to improve ECG recording with the capillary electrometer, but he became increasingly frustrated with the device's limitations. The capillary electrometer was slow to react to changes in current, and was very sensitive to interference from nearby sources of vibration.

It was only with Einthoven's invention of a string galvanometer at the turn of the century that high-quality ECG recording became possible. Einthoven's string galvanometer consisted of a fine quartz thread, coated in silver, strung between the poles of a magnet. The thread was created by dipping an arrow into molten glass and then firing it across the laboratory, drawing the glass out into an extremely fine thread. Variations in current caused the thread to vibrate, and the movements of the thread were magnified and recorded upon photographic paper.

Einthoven's string galvanometer, despite its sensitivity, was a very large and cumbersome device – it filled two rooms, the electromagnet had a tendency to overheat, and the subject from whom the ECG was recorded had to sit with hands and feet in buckets of saline. Nevertheless, the clinical usefulness of the device rapidly became clear and a telephone cable was laid to connect the apparatus in Einthoven's laboratory to the local hospital over a kilometre away! Einthoven's invention led to him being awarded the Nobel Prize in 1924.

● Development of commercial ECG machines

Within a decade of Einthoven's publication of the first string galvanometer ECG recordings in 1902, a commercial ECG machine based on his invention became available. Einthoven worked with the Cambridge Scientific Instrument Company to refine his invention and to produce a marketable ECG machine.

The company's very first version of Einthoven's machine, much reduced in size, was launched in 1908. A table-sized version was subsequently developed, and the first of these machines was delivered to Sir Thomas Lewis (who himself would have a major role in developing the clinical application of electrocardiography). It was not until 1926 that a portable ECG machine was launched. Weighing in at 36 kg (80 lb), it was still a cumbersome device, but was nonetheless a major step forwards in making ECG recording more widely available.

● ECG nomenclature

In his early ECG recordings, Waller named the waveforms he observed ABCD (four deflections were recognized at that time). Mathematical techniques (using differential equations) were subsequently used to improve the quality of ECG recordings. It was traditional that mathematical notation used letters from the latter half of the alphabet. Curved lines were traditionally labelled starting at P, and straight lines starting at Q. Hence the familiar PQRST notation was introduced to label the deflections on the ECG, and was used for the first time by Einthoven.

The use of the chest leads was first described in the 1930s, and at around the same time Frank Wilson invented the 'indifferent electrode' (also known as the 'Wilson central terminal'). This led to the development of the 'unipolar' limb leads VR, VL and VF (with the letter 'V' standing for 'voltage'). In 1942 the American cardiologist Emanuel Goldberger increased the voltage of these leads by 50 per cent, leading to the term 'augmented' leads (aVR, aVL and aVF). By this stage the 12-lead ECG which remains familiar today finally took shape, and its format has remained essentially unchanged since that time.

● Ambulatory ECG monitoring

Ambulatory ECG monitoring – the ability to record the ECG while the patient is active – is invaluable in the diagnosis of episodic palpitations. Its origins lie in the work of Norman J Holter, and ambulatory recorders are often referred to as Holter monitors in recognition of his key contributions to this field. In the 1950s he described the technique of 'radioelectrocardiography', in which an

ECG recording could be transmitted by telemetry from a transmitter carried by the patient to a base station. His original device weighed 38.5 kg (85 lb) and was worn as a back pack! As the technique was refined and equipment became more portable, the ability to record the ECG signal was incorporated into the device, so that a 24-h recording could be made using a tape within the unit carried by the patient. In recent years, further miniaturization of electronic components and the introduction of solid-state digital recording media have further reduced the size of ambulatory ECG recorders and improved the duration and quality of recordings.

Further reading

If you would like to know more about the history of the ECG, the following textbook and website are particularly informative:

Acierno LJ. *The History of Cardiology*. London: Taylor and Francis, 1994. (ISBN 978-1850703396) *An excellent and extremely detailed history of cardiology.*

ECG Library. A (not so) brief history of electrocardiography. Available at www.ecglibrary.com/ecghist.html (accessed August 2007).

Useful websites and further reading

● Useful websites

The following websites are particularly useful for anyone wanting to learn more about ECG interpretation:

ECG Library: www.ecglibrary.com

The Alan E Lindsay ECG Learning Center: http://library.med. utah.edu/kw/ecg

The Six Second ECG. Dynamic Cardiac Rhythm Simulator: www.skillstat.com/Flash/ECGSim531.html

(All websites accessed August 2007.)

● ECG interpretation and arrhythmias

Bennett DH. *Cardiac Arrhythmias*, 7th edn. London: Hodder Arnold, 2006. (ISBN 978-0340925621) An excellent guide to the diagnosis and treatment of cardiac arrhythmias.

Azeem T, Vassallo M, Samani N. *Rapid Review of ECG Interpretation*. London: Manson Publishing, 2005. (ISBN 978-1840760439) A good case-based approach to ECG interpretation.

Springhouse. *ECG Interpretation Made Incredibly Easy*, 3rd edn. Philadelphia: Lippincott Williams & Wilkins, 2004. (ISBN 978-1582553559). A good and very readable introductory textbook.

● Cardiology textbooks

Grubb NR, Newby DE. *Churchill's Pocketbook of Cardiology*, 2nd edn. Edinburgh: Churchill Livingstone, 2006. (ISBN 978-0443100512) A detailed and up-to-date pocket-sized handbook of cardiology.

Julian DG, Campbell-Cowan J, McLenachan JM. *Cardiology*, 8th edn. Edinburgh: Saunders, 2004. (ISBN 978-0702026959) A useful handbook of cardiovascular medicine.

● Resuscitation guidelines

In the UK, the teaching of advanced life support is coordinated nationally by the Resuscitation Council (UK).

Resuscitation Council (UK)
5th Floor, Tavistock House North
Tavistock Square
London WC1H 9HR
United Kingdom

Tel: 020 7388 4678
Fax: 020 7383 0773
Email: enquiries@resus.org.uk
Website: www.resus.org.uk

The European Resuscitation Council Guidelines for Resuscitation 2005 can be found in the following journal:

European Resuscitation Council. European Resuscitation Council Guidelines for Resuscitation 2005. *Resuscitation* 2005; **67**(Suppl 1):S1–S190.

Help with the next edition

We would like to know what you would like to see included (or omitted!) in the next edition of *Making Sense of the ECG*. Please send your comments or suggestions to:

Dr Andrew R Houghton
Making Sense of the ECG
c/o Hodder Arnold, Health Sciences
338 Euston Road
London NW1 3BH

We will include acknowledgements to all those whose suggestions are used in the next edition.

Index

ABCDE approach 253
ABCDEF mnemonic 267
accelerated idioventricular rhythm
    25, 56
accessory pathways
    ablation 52
    and AV re-entry tachycardia 47,
        48, 49, 52
    and axis deviation 96, 98
    of Lown–Ganong–Levine
        syndrome 117
    of Wolff–Parkinson–White
        syndrome 48, 96, 98,
        114–16, 142
accident and emergency departments
    235
acid-base abnormalities 57
acidaemia 257
acute coronary syndrome 187,
    189–90
    non-ST segment elevation 160,
        179
    ST segment elevation 159–69, 180
adenosine 23, 39–40, 51–2, 265
adrenaline 33, 255, 257, 258, 263
agonal breaths 253
airway assessment 252, 253–4, 266
albumin 209, 216
alcohol 33, 41
alpha receptors 172
ALS (Advanced Life Support) 66,
    251, 255–8
ambulances 252

ambulatory ECG recording 26,
    232–8, 271–2
    24hr (Holter monitor) 37, 232–4
    bedside monitoring/telemetry
        (inpatient) 232–3, 236–7
    ECG 'on demand' 232–3, 235–6
    for ectopic beats 64
    event recorders 232–3, 234–5
    implantable loop recorder 232–3,
        237–8
    for sick sinus syndrome 37
aminophylline 263
amiodarone
    in atrial fibrillation 46, 52, 264
    in atrial flutter 41, 264
    in ventricular fibrillation 58,
        255
    in ventricular tachycardia 54, 55,
        265
amyloidosis 37
anaemia 33
anaesthesia, general 45
analgesia 179
aneurysm 241
    left ventricular 159, 169–70
aneurysmectomy 170
angina 161, 197
    atypical 247
    Prinzmetal's (vasospastic) 159,
        170–2
    stable 177–8, 239
    typical 247, 249
    unstable 159, 160

angiotensin-converting enzyme (ACE) inhibitors 168, 178
anterior fascicle 11, 13, 92–5, 93
  see also left anterior hemiblock
anti-anginal treatment 178, 241
anti-arrhythmic drugs 57, 64, 170, 180–2, 209
  contraindications 46
  see also specific drugs
anti-emetics 167
anti-inflammatories 173
antibiotics 211
anticoagulation 42, 44, 45, 170
  contraindications to 46
antidepressants, tricyclic 209
antiplatelet drugs 42
aorta, coarctation 139
aortic dissection 162
aortic stenosis 139, 152, 240, 241
apex beat 142, 145
appropriate discordance 175
arrhythmia 19, 23
  and acute myocarditis 210–11
  categorization 29
  diagnosis 258–61
  and digoxin toxicity 181
  exercise-related 239, 241, 243
  and hyperkalaemia 188, 189
  identification 28–9
  and left ventricular aneurysm 170
  management 250, 255–61
  mis-diagnosis 250
  'non-shockable' 255, 256, 257–8
  'shockable' 255–7, 258
  ventricular 25, 184, 211–12, 230, 243
  of Wolff–Parkinson–White syndrome 116
  see also specific arrhythmias
arrhythmogenic right ventricular cardiomyopathy (ARVC) 54, 55
artefacts 217–21
arterial blood gases 267
aspirin 44, 161, 167, 168, 177, 179
AST (aspartate transaminase) 162–3
asystole 22, 67, 74, 102, 184
  diagnosis 258, 259–60

management 161, 229, 255, 258, 259–60, 262–3
  predictors of 264
atherosclerosis 170
atrial activity
  assessment 71–2
  independent 75, 76, 105
  unclear 72
  and ventricular activity 72–4
  see also atrial depolarization
atrial depolarization 7, 9, 18
  abnormal 106–7
  assessment 71–3
  axis for 92
  duration 3
  erratic 42, 43
  and the P wave 3, 9, 18, 71, 100, 101, 102
  and the PR interval 113
atrial ectopics 61, 107
atrial fibrillation 23–4, 36, 42–6, 68, 71–2, 77
  with aberrant conduction 265
  in congenital short QT syndromes 204
  in hypothermia 184
  idiopathic ('lone') 41
  management 44–6, 47, 52, 264
  and the P wave 102
  and pacing 229
  paroxysmal 42, 46
  permanent 42, 43
  persistent 42
  with pre-excitation 265
  prevention of spread 10
  and pulseless electrical activity 261
  recurrent 45, 46
  resistant 47
  in Wolff–Parkinson–White syndrome 52
atrial flutter 24, 36, 39–42, 71
  ablation 42
  causes 40–1
  management 40–2, 45
  misdiagnosis 33–4
  P waves in 105
atrial kick, loss of 43

atrial myocardial remodelling 47
atrial rate 21, 40
atrial rhythm 30, 37–46, 66, 124
atrial septal defect 41, 152
atrial tachycardia 24, 36, 37–9, 77
  with AV block 181, 264
  misdiagnosis 33–4
  paroxysmal 181
atrioventricular node (AV) *see* AV node
atrium 9–10, 65
  accessory pathways 114–15
  and AV re-entry tachycardias 46
  left enlargement 46, 109
  and pacemakers 227
  right 9, 39
  right enlargement 107–9
atropine 23, 33, 258, 263
autosomal dominant disorders
    204–5, 211
autosomal recessive disorders 211
AV block 38, 58, 181, 184
  2:1 39, 40, 120, 122–3
  3:1 39, 40
  4:1 39, 40
  in atrial flutter 39–40, 41
  congenital 125, 225
  first-degree 58, 95, 118–19, 215
  intermittent 68
  Mobitz type I (Wenckebach
    phenomenon) 119, 225
  Mobitz type II 120, 121–2, 225,
    264
  second-degree 22, 39–40, 58,
    119–25, 229, 264
  third-degree (complete) 22, 58–9,
    73, 94, 120, 122–5, 224–5,
    229, 263
AV dissociation 73–4, 125
AV junction 65, 69
  bypass 113, 114–15, 117
  depolarization originating in the
    113–14
  and pacing 228
  and the PR interval 112, 113
  as regulator of conduction 112,
    113
AV junctional ectopics 61–2, 114
AV junctional pacemaker 59–60

AV junctional rhythm 30, 107
AV junctional tachycardia 103–4,
  107
AV nodal blocking drugs 43, 52
AV nodal conduction disorders 36,
  78, 118
AV nodal escape rhythms 114
AV nodal pathways, dual 47–9
AV nodal re-entry tachycardia 33,
  48–51, 72, 77, 265
AV node 9–10, 18, 112, 114
  ablation 47
  atrial depolarization from a focus
    near the 71, 72, 106–7
  in atrial fibrillation 42
  rhythm 113
  and ventricular depolarization 70
AV node block 51
AV re-entry circuit 46–8
AV re-entry tachycardia 24, 30,
  46–52, 77, 114, 261, 265
axis, cardiac 31, 80–99
  definition 80–1, 84
  left axis deviation 87–8, 92–6,
    138, 155
  and the limb leads 82–91
  measurement 80–92
  normal 86–8, 89
  range of angles 82–3
  reference/zero point 82
  right axis deviation 87–8, 91,
    96–8, 139, 140, 142, 155

back pain 162
Bazett's formula 202, 203
Beck's triad 145
bedrest 179, 210
bedside monitoring/telemetry
  232–3, 236–7
beta blockers 23, 32, 264
  in atrial fibrillation 43
  in atrial flutter 40
  in atrial tachycardia 38
  in AV block 118
  drug interactions 39, 44, 52
  in myocardial ischaemia 178, 179
  in Prinzmetal's angina 172
  in sick sinus syndrome 37

beta blockers (*contd*)
  in sinus tachycardia 33, 34
  in ST segment elevation acute
      coronary syndrome 168
  in ventricular fibrillation 58
bifascicular block 93–5, 225, 229
bigeminy 62, 63, 68, 181
bisphosphonates 206
black people, T wave inversion 193
blood glucose 267
blood pressure
  and exercise ECG testing 241, 242,
      243, 244
  systolic 243, 244, 263
  see also hypertension; hypotension
BLS (basic life support) 57, 251–2
Borrelia burgdorferi 125
bradycardia 21–4, 27, 67
  and AV block 120, 124
  management 23–4, 222–6,
      229–30, 258, 263–4
  pacing 222–6, 229–30
  peri-arrest 263–4
  vagally induced 118
  see also sinus bradycardia;
      tachycardia–bradycardia
      (tachy–brady) syndrome
breathing assessment 252, 253, 266
breathlessness 145, 243
bronchitis, chronic 109
Bruce protocol 241, 242
Brugada syndrome 159, 176
buccal nitrate 178, 179
bundle branch block 58, 59, 172
  exercise-induced 244
  incomplete 153, 154–5
  left 55, 59, 64, 69, 75, 94, 129
    and acute myocardial infarction
        160
    causes 152
    and exercise ECG testing 241
    incomplete 154
    and the QRS complex 146,
        147–52
    and ST segment elevation 159,
        160, 168, 175
  management 265
  pre-existing/rate-dependent 50

  right 59, 69, 75, 93–5, 97, 129,
      136, 139
    in Brugada syndrome 176
    causes 152
    and exercise ECG testing 241
    incomplete 154–5
    and the QRS complex 146, 147,
        148–52
  and the T wave 194
bundle branches 224
  left 10–11, 13, 59, 92, 124, 136,
      147, 154
  right 10–11, 59, 92, 124, 147,
      154
bundle of His 10–11, 48–9, 69–70
  and AV block 121, 123–4
  and the bundle of James 117
  conduction through 112, 114
bundle of James 117
bundle of Kent 114, 117, 142
Burdon Sanderson, John 269

caffeine 26, 33
calcium
  intravenous/oral 209
  plasma levels 205, 206, 208, 216
calcium antagonists 23
calcium-channel blockers 118, 172,
    178
calibration 17, 19, 136, 143
  incorrect 217, 218
calibration mark 17, 219
capillary electrometer 269–70
capture beats 75, 76, 77
cardiac arrest 54, 206, 255–8
  aftercare 266–7
  management 254, 255–8, 266–7
  peri-arrest arrhythmias 263–5
  reversible causes 257
  rhythms 74
cardiac catheterization 178, 179
cardiac death, sudden 57, 176, 204,
    209
cardiac magnetic resonance imaging
    55, 132
cardiac markers 159, 160, 162–3,
    210
  serial measurements 131

cardiac output 43, 263
cardiac (pericardial) tamponade 145, 146, 257
cardiac resynchronization treatment 231
cardiac risk factors 161–2
cardiac transplantation 170
cardiomyopathy 37, 38, 41, 152
  arrhythmogenic right ventricular 54–5
  dilated 54
  hypertrophic 54, 139, 207
  hypertrophic obstructive 240, 241
  ischaemic 230
cardiopulmonary resuscitation (CPR) 241, 250–67
  advanced life support (ALS) 66, 251, 255–8
  aftercare 266–7
  arrhythmia diagnosis 258–61
  basic life support (BLS) 57, 251–2
  chain of survival 251
  defibrillator use 251, 261–2
  directing others during the arrest 266
  early intervention 251
  inhospital resuscitation 252–4
  peri-arrest arrhythmias 263–5
  training 250–1
carotid bruits 40, 51
carotid pulse 253, 254
carotid sinus massage 39–41, 51, 265
carotid sinus syndrome 226
cerebral injury 207
cerebral thromboembolism 40
chest compressions 252–4, 257, 258, 266
chest pain 51, 162, 171, 179, 197, 243, 247
  diagnosis 239
  tight, central 161
chest radiography 109, 142, 146, 162, 170, 210, 225, 267
chronic obstructive pulmonary disease 38
Chvostek's sign 208
CK-MB 162–3

clinical context 66
clopidogrel 167, 168, 179
colchicine 173
conduction 69–70
  accelerated 65
  anterograde 46, 48
  normal 65
  retrograde 46, 48, 62, 105, 107
conduction disturbances 30, 58–9, 65, 68–70, 73, 75, 93–5, 171–2, 243
  AV 119–25
  see also specific disturbances
conduction system 69–70
  fibrosis of the 92, 93, 152
congenital heart disease 54, 125, 204–5, 225
congenital high-tone deafness 211
congenital long QT syndromes 57
congenital short QT syndromes 204–5
connective tissue disease 173
Cornell criteria 137
coronary angiography 132, 167
coronary artery, right 171
coronary artery bypass surgery 178
coronary artery disease 45, 177, 180
  and exercise ECG testing 241, 244–7, 249
  risk factors for 162, 244, 247, 249
coronary care unit 163
corticosteroids, systemic 173
cosine 90–1
creatine kinase (CK) 162

DC cardioversion 26, 262
  in atrial fibrillation 44–5, 46, 52
  in atrial flutter 42, 45
  in AV re-entry tachycardias 52
  low-energy shocks 55
  in peri-arrest tachycardia 264
  in supraventricular tachycardia 75
  in ventricular fibrillation 57
  in ventricular tachycardia 54, 75, 265
deafness, congenital high-tone 211

defibrillation 45, 254, 255, 261–2, 266
  biphasic defibrillators 45, 262
  visual sweeps 262
  see also implantable cardioverter defibrillators
deflection
  direction 5, 6–7
  equipolar 6
  intrinsicoid 138
  negative 5, 6–7, 9, 84, 86, 87–90
  positive 5, 6–7, 9, 84–90
delta wave 51, 115–16, 134, 155–6
depolarization 2
  and AV junctional bypasses 113, 114–15, 117
  axis of 81, 84, 92, 96
  and hyperkalaemia 146
  originating in the AV junction 113–14
  pacing and 227
  septal 11, 128
  wave of 9–13
  see also atrial depolarization; ventricular depolarization
dextrocardia 96, 98, 106, 136, 142–3
diabetes 44, 162
diagnostic software 237, 238
diathermy 42, 229
digoxin 23, 32, 37, 264
  in atrial fibrillation 43, 45, 46
  in atrial flutter 40
  in AV block 118
  plasma levels 182
  and the QT interval 204, 206–7
  and ST segment depression 177, 180–2
  and the T wave 194, 198–9
  toxicity 38, 45, 181–2, 194, 198–9, 207, 241
diuretics 192
  potassium-sparing 188
  thiazide 206
dizziness 23, 25, 37, 51, 54, 125, 243
dopamine 263
double impulse 170
Dressler's syndrome 173

drug histories 23
drug-induced pericarditis 173
drug interactions 57
drugs 37, 46
  in AV block 118
  in AV re-entry tachycardia 51–2
  and the QT interval 206–7, 209–10
  and ST segment depression 177, 180–2
  in ventricular tachycardia 54–5
  see also specific drugs
dual AV nodal pathways 47–9
dyslipidaemia 162

early intervention 251
Ebstein's anomaly 152
ECG 'on demand' 232–3, 235–6
ECG rulers 20
echocardiography 43, 55, 64, 109, 132, 139, 146, 170
ectopic beats (extrasystoles/premature beats) 30, 61–4, 68–9
  atrial 61, 107
  AV junctional 61–2, 114
  prevention 47
  'R on T' 62
  ventricular 55, 61–4, 68–70, 107, 153, 181
Einthoven, Willem 269–70, 271
electrical alternans 145
electrical impulses
  direction of flow through the heart 5, 6–7, 80–2, 84–92
  see also depolarization; repolarization
electrical interference, external 217, 218–19
electrodes 229
  assessment 67
  chest 4, 17, 144
  correct position 17, 106
  disconnection 67
  limb 4–5, 17
  misplacement 217–18
electrolyte levels 45, 206, 267
  imbalances 32, 54, 57

electromechanical dissociation *see* pulseless electrical activity
electrophysiological studies (EPS) 230
embolism 170
　systemic 43
　see also pulmonary embolism; thromboembolism
embolization 46
emphysema 109, 143–4
escape beats 32, 35, 36
escape rhythms 22, 30, 59–61, 102
　AV junctional 22
　in sick sinus syndrome 36, 37
　in sinus bradycardia 32
　ventricular 22
event recorders 232–3, 234–5
exercise ECG testing 64, 132, 177, 239–49
　Bruce protocol 241, 242
　contraindications to 240, 241
　interpretation 243–9
　metabolic equivalents 242
　modified Bruce protocol 241, 242
　process 240–2
　prognostic nomogram for 248, 249
　risks 240
　stopping 242–3
exercise tolerance 239
exhaustion 243

F (fibrillation) wave 42, 71, 72, 102
F (flutter) wave 39–40, 41, 71, 105
fascicular block 59, 92–5, 153, 155, 172
　see also bifascicular block; trifascicular block
fatigue 243
fever 210, 240
fibrosis
　of the conduction system 92, 93, 152
　of the SA node 37
flat line 67, 260
flecainide 41, 46, 54, 209
fluid balance 168, 267
fluid loss 33
frail patients 241

friction rub 173, 210
full blood count 267
furosemide 206
fusion beats 75, 76

gain setting 67, 219
gallop rhythm 210
gastrocnemius muscle 268
gel pads 262
gene mutations 204, 211
glyceryl trinitrate 177, 241
glycoprotein IIb/IIIa inhibitors 179
Goldberger, Emanuel 271
Goswell, Thomas 269

haemodynamic disturbance 29, 168
　and AV block 120, 124–5
　and bradycardia 23, 24
　and pacing 224
　and pericardial effusion 146
　and tachycardia 26, 53, 54, 259
haemorrhage 194, 260
heart block 32, 210–11
　first-degree 191
　see also specific blocks
heart failure 33, 125, 170, 210–11, 263
　and atrial fibrillation 44
　management 222, 231
　right 168
　uncontrolled 240
heart rate 19–27
　in accelerated idioventricular rhythm 56
　atrial 21, 38, 40
　in AV nodal re-entry tachycardias/AV re-entry tachycardias 49–50
　bradycardic 21, 31
　electrical basis 268
　escape rhythms 60
　in exercise ECG testing 242–3
　irregular 20
　measurement 19–21
　normal 9, 21
　and the QT interval 202, 203
　regular 19–20
　in sinus arrhythmia 31, 32–3, 34

heart rate (*contd*)
  in sinus rhythm 30, 31
  tachycardic 21, 24–6, 32–3, 34,
    38, 53
  ventricular 19, 39, 45–6, 53, 67,
    263
  zero 22
heart sounds
  fourth 170, 210
  quiet 210
  soft 145
heparin 179
high take-off (early repolarization)
  159, 174
His–Purkinje conduction system
  69–70
history of the ECG 268–72
Holter monitoring 37, 232–4
Holter, Norman J 271–2
hypercalcaemia 204, 205–6, 214,
  216
hyperkalaemia 103, 146, 187–9, 257
hyperparathyroidism 206
hypertension 41, 139, 152, 162
  and atrial fibrillation 44
  pulmonary 109, 140, 241
  uncontrolled 240
hyperthermia 204
hyperthyroidism 33, 41, 214, 216
hyperventilation 194
hypocalaemia 207, 208–9, 257
hypokalaemia 118, 190, 191–2, 214,
  215, 257
hypoparathyroidism 209
hypotension 145, 168, 224
hypothermia 32, 183–4, 207, 257
hypothyroidism 32, 190, 192
hypovolaemia 257
hypoxia 257

implantable cardioverter
    defibrillators (ICDs) 55, 57,
    64, 204, 212, 222, 230
implantable loop recorders 232–3,
  237–8
inappropriate concordance 175
infections 173, 210
inspiration 34, 128, 129, 173, 193

international normalized ratio
  (INR) 45
interventricular septum 10–11, 15,
  18, 92, 133, 147, 148, 224
intracranial pressure 32
intravenous access 266
intravenous fluids 168
intubation 266
ischaemic heart disease 32–3, 37–8,
  41, 54, 118, 132, 152, 230
  exercise ECG testing for 239, 243
  risk factors 162, 197
  and the ST segment 15
  see also myocardial ischaemia
isoelectric deflections 84, 85, 87
isoprenaline 263
ivabradine 178

J point 244
J wave (Osborn wave) 183–4
jaundice, obstructive 32
Jervell and Lange-Nielsen syndrome
  211
jugular venous pressure 145
junctional escape beat 35

lactate dehydrogenase (LDH) 162–3
leads 4–8
  bipolar 4
  chest 4, 5–6, 271
  limb 4–5, 271
  names 4
  nomenclature 4
  number of 4, 7
  unipolar 4
  viewpoints 4–6, 7
left anterior hemiblock 92–5, 98
left atrial enlargement 46, 109
left axis deviation 87–8, 92–6, 138,
  155
left bundle branch block *see* bundle
  branch block, left
left cervical sympathectomy 57
left posterior hemiblock 96, 98
left ventricle 11–12
left ventricular aneurysm 159,
  169–70
left ventricular ejection fraction 231

left ventricular hypertrophy *see* ventricular hypertrophy, left
Lewis, Sir Thomas 270–1
lidocaine (lignocaine) 54, 58
life support 57, 66, 251–2, 255–8
Lippmann, Gabriel 269
long QT syndrome (LQTS) 54, 57, 207, 211–12
Lown–Ganong–Levine (LGL) syndrome 113, 117–18
Lyme disease 118, 125

magnesium 57
magnesium sulphate 265
malignancy 173, 206
malignant vasovagal syndrome 226
Marey, Étienne-Jules 269
metabolic equivalents (METs) 242
milk-alkali syndrome 206
millivolts 2–3
misdiagnosis 16, 33, 66
mitral stenosis 46
mitral valve disease 109
mitral valve prolapse 54, 194
Muirhead, Alexander 269
Müller, Heinrich 268
myocardial infarction 32, 93, 159
  acute 33, 54, 55, 56, 57, 160
    anterior 7, 8, 120, 124, 190, 224
    and AV block 120–1, 122, 124
    and bundle branch block 150
    inferior 7, 8, 120, 124, 131, 224
    management 224, 225
    posterior 177, 179, 189
    and QT interval 207
  anterior 7, 8, 120, 124, 130, 165, 190, 224
  anterolateral 96, 98
  and exercise ECG testing 239, 240, 241
  inferior 7, 8, 92, 96, 120, 124, 131, 224
  large 260
  lateral 164
  non-ST segment elevation 160
  posterior 136, 139–41, 177, 179, 189

right ventricular 168
risk stratification 239
silent/painless 132
and ST segment elevation 15, 129, 130–3, 160, 161–5, 168, 169, 173, 175
and the T wave 194, 196–7
myocardial ischaemia 175, 177–80, 194–5, 263
myocardial necrosis 132, 159, 160, 162
myocardial reperfusion 167
myocarditis 37, 41, 54
  acute 207, 210–11, 240
  rheumatic 118
myocytes 153
  necrosis markers 159, 160, 162

National Institute for Health and Clinical Excellence (NICE) 31
  AF management guidelines 44
nausea 161
necrosis, myocardial 132, 159, 160, 162
negatively chronotropic drugs 23, 32
neurological status 267
nicorandil 178
'nil by mouth' 45
nitrate 172, 177, 178, 179, 241
non-ST segment elevation acute coronary syndrome (NSTEACS) 160, 179
non-ST segment elevation myocardial infarction (NSTEMI) 160, 196, 197
nuclear myocardial perfusion scan 132

obesity 92, 143–4, 162
overdrive pacing 32, 52, 54, 55, 224
overweight 162
oxygen therapy 167, 253

P wave 2, 58, 72–4
  absent 101–5
  assessment 100–11
  in asystole 67, 259–60

P wave (*contd*)
  in atrial depolarization 3, 9, 18,
        71, 100, 101, 102
  in atrial fibrillation 42, 43
  in atrial tachycardia 37, 38
  in AV block 119–24
  in AV nodal re-entry
        tachycardias/AV re-entry
        tachycardias 49, 50
  and the axis 92
  bifid 109–10
  biphasic 105–6
  in capture beats 77
  definition 9, 18
  in ectopic beats 61–2, 63
  flattening and loss 188
  and the heart rate 21
  in independent atrial activity 75,
        76
  interval between subsequent
        waves 10
  inversion 7, 71, 105–7, 142
  normal 107, 109
  orientation 7
  origin 100
  in P mitrale 109–10
  in P pulmonale 107–9
  pacing and 228
  in sick sinus syndrome 35, 36
  in sinus arrhythmia 34
  in sinus bradycardia 31
  in sinus rhythm 30, 31
  in sinus tachycardia 32–3
  tall 107–9
  upright 7
  wide 109–10
  width 3
pacemakers of the heart
  SA node 101, 105, 106
  subsidiary 59–60, 123–4
  ventricular 31, 60
pacing 61, 222–9
  AAI 227
  AAIR 227
  for atrial fibrillation 47
  for AV block 120–1, 122, 124–5
  awaiting permanent 223
  batteries 223

  biventricular 231
  for bradycardia 23–4
  codes 226
  DDD 227
  DDDR 227
  dual-chamber sequential 22
  and the ECG 227–9
  emergency 67
  function 222–3
  insertion 224–5
  overdrive 32, 52, 54, 55, 224
  percussion 67, 223
  perioperative 229
  permanent 47, 94–5, 125, 194,
        223, 225–7, 229, 230, 239
  prophylactic 120–1
  rate-responsive 227
  for sick sinus syndrome 37
  and surgery 229
  temporary 57, 120–1, 124–5,
        223–5, 229
  transcutaneous 67, 223, 263
  transoesophageal 223
  transvenous 67, 223, 263
  ventricular 31, 47, 60, 194, 227–8
  for ventricular tachycardia 54, 55
  VVI 227
  VVIR 227
pacing 'spikes' 227–9
pacing wire 224–5
Page, Frederick 269
pain
  back 162
  retrosternal 173
  see also chest pain
pain relief 167
  see also anaesthesia; analgesia
palpitations 25, 37, 43, 51, 54, 116,
        210, 271
  obtaining ECG readings during
        232–6
  'tapping out' 25
pancreatitis, acute 209
paper speed 3, 17, 19
  incorrect 217, 220
papilloedema 208
patient histories 25
patient movement 217, 220–1

percutaneous coronary intervention (PCI) 167, 178
peri-arrest arrhythmias 263–5
pericardial aspiration 146
pericardial (cardiac) tamponade 145, 146, 257
pericardial effusion 144–6, 190, 192
pericarditis 41, 159, 172–3
  acute 240
  drug-induced 173
  and the T wave 194
peripheral perfusion 267
physical inactivity 162
pneumonia 41
pneumothorax 225, 257
positively chronotropic drugs 26, 33
posterior fascicle 11, 13, 92–5
potassium channels 211
potassium chloride 192
potassium plasma levels 45, 103, 182
  elevated 103, 146, 187–9, 257
  low 118, 190, 191–2, 214, 215, 257
potassium supplements 188
PR interval 112–26
  assessment 113–26
  in atrioventricular block 58, 94
  in AV nodal re-entry
      tachycardias/AV re-entry
      tachycardias 51
  definition 10, 18, 112
  greater than 0.2s long (prolonged) 58, 94, 118–19
  lengthening 188
  of less than 0.12s long 113–18, 142, 156
  unmeasurable 119–25
  variable 119–25
precordial thump 254
pregnancy 92
presyncope 225, 229
Prinzmetal's (vasospastic) angina 159, 170–2
pro-arrhythmic drugs 54
procainamide 209
pseudohypoparathyroidism 209
pulmonary embolism 33, 41, 194
  massive 109, 152, 197, 260
  and Q waves 129

pulmonary hypertension 109, 140, 241
pulmonary stenosis 109, 140
pulmonary vein isolation 47
pulse
  carotid 253, 254
  checking for 257
  irregularly irregular 43
pulseless electrical activity (PEA) 66, 74
  diagnosis 258, 260–1
  management 255, 257–8, 260–1, 262
pulseless ventricular fibrillation 258
pulseless ventricular tachycardia
  diagnosis 259
  management 255–7, 259, 261
pulsus paradoxus 145
Purkinje fibres 11–12, 69–70, 114, 153

Q wave 2, 8, 10, 11, 12, 141
  in bundle branch block 147, 148
  definition 127
  in myocardial infarction 161
  narrow 129, 193
  normal 128–9
  pathological 127–34, 193
  in pericarditis 173
  septal 128, 133, 148
  in ST segment elevation acute
      coronary syndrome 160, 196
  wide 129
QRS complex 11–14, 135–57, 269
  abnormally shaped 153–6
  in accelerated idioventricular
      rhythm 56
  assessment 67–73, 75
  in atrial fibrillation 42, 43, 68, 102
  in atrial flutter 39, 40, 41
  in AV block 119–24
  in AV nodal re-entry
      tachycardias/AV re-entry
      tachycardias 49–50
  and the axis 80, 84–90, 93, 98

QRS complex (*contd*)
  broad 24–5, 50, 53, 56, 60, 62,
       63, 66, 69–71, 75, 124,
       136, 146–53, 175, 184,
       227–8
  buried P waves on 105
  in capture beats 77
  in conductance disturbance 68
  definition 18
  in ectopic beats 61–2, 63
  equipolar 13
  in escape rhythms 59, 60
  first part of the 115
  and heart rate 19–21
  hidden 72
  and incorrect calibration 219
  in left bundle branch block 175
  missed 68
  narrow 24, 50, 62, 70–1, 123
  negative 11–14
  normal 135, 136, 143, 146
  notched 153, 155, 175
  oversized R waves 135, 136–42
  oversized S waves 135, 136–42
  and pacing 227–8, 231
  positive 11–14
  Q waves and 127
  regularity 67–8
  in sinus arrhythmia 34
  in sinus bradycardia 31
  in sinus rhythm 30, 31
  slurred 153, 155–6
  small 142–6, 192
  in tachycardia 24–5, 32–3, 53, 78,
       105
  in torsades de pointes 56
  types 11–12
  widening 188
QT interval 57, 181, 201–12
  calculation 202
  definition 15, 18, 201
  normal 201–3
  overestimation 202
  too long 184, 202, 207–12
  too short 202, 204–7
quinidine 37
  and AV block 118
  and the QT interval 209

and ST segment depression 177,
       180, 182

'R on T' ectopics 62
R wave 2, 10–14, 189
  and the axis 89, 97
  in bundle branch block 147–8,
       150–1
  dominant 139–40, 179
  normal 136
  oversized 135, 136–43, 180,
       182–3, 197
  in pericardial effusion 145
  and Q waves 128
  R' 147
  in ventricular hypertrophy 197
radioelectrocardiography 271–2
radiofrequency ablation 52
radiotherapy 173
Raynaud's phenomenon 171
recording ECGs 16–18
relaxation 2
renal failure, chronic 209
repolarization 2, 15
  abnormalities following
       paroxysmal tachycardia 194
  and appropriate discordance 175
  early 159, 174
  see also ventricular repolarization
rescue breaths 252
respiratory arrest 254
resting ECG, abnormal 241
Resuscitation Council (UK) 66,
       250–1
retrosternal pain 173
return of spontaneous circulation
       (ROSC) 266
rheumatic carditis 210
rheumatic heart disease 38, 41, 118,
       210
rheumatic myocarditis 118
rhythm 28–79
  atrial 30, 37–46, 66, 124
  AV junctional 30, 107
  common 29–64
  conduction 65
  identification 64–78
  monitoring 267

normal 29–31
source of the 65, 69
see also specific rhythms
rhythm strips 28
right atrial enlargement (P pulmonale) 107–9
right atrium 9, 39
right axis deviation 87–8, 91, 96–8, 139, 140, 142, 155
right bundle branch block *see* bundle branch block, right
right ventricular hypertrophy *see* ventricular hypertrophy, right
right ventricular outflow tract (RVOT) tachycardia 55, 64
Romano–Ward syndrome 211
Romhilt-Estes scoring system 137–9
RR interval 202, 203
RS complexes 49

S wave 2, 11–15
and the axis 89, 97
in bundle branch block 147–8, 150–1
and high take-off 174
normal 136
oversized 135, 136–42, 182–3, 197
SA arrest 59
SA block 22, 35–6, 58–9, 72
P waves in 100, 102, 105
SA nodal rhythms 29–37
SA node 65
and atrial activity 71, 73
degeneration and fibrosis 37
depolarization 9, 10, 18, 100
electrophysiological modification/ablation 34
pacemaker function 101, 105, 106
and sinus rhythm 29
and ventricular activity 73
salbutamol 33
saline 206
sarcoidosis 206
'sawtooth' baselines 39–40, 71, 105
sciatic nerve 268
septal depolarization 11, 128
sick sinus syndrome 22, 32, 35–7, 38, 41

causes 37
management 37, 226
signal-averaged ECGs 221
sine 90–1
sinoatrial node *see* SA node
sinus arrest 22, 35, 72, 102–3, 105
sinus arrhythmia 34–5, 68, 101
sinus bradycardia 22, 31–2, 59, 181
and hypothyroidism 192
of sick sinus syndrome 35
sinus rhythm 29–31, 231
induction 261
P waves in 101, 103
restoration 41, 43, 44–5, 46
sinus tachycardia 24, 32–4, 77, 265
appropriate 33
inappropriate 33–4
management 33–4
P waves in 104
persistent 33–4
skeletal muscle activity 220–1
smoking 162
sodium channels 176, 211
$S_IQ_{III}T_{III}$ pattern 129
sotalol 41, 46, 52, 54, 55
ST segment 104, 158–85
in acute myocarditis 210
definition 15, 18
depression 139–41, 160, 166, 172, 175–84, 189, 191, 197, 215, 243–5, 247, 249
elevated 8, 141, 159–76, 179
and exercise testing 243, 244–5, 247, 249
in hyperkalaemia 188
isoelectric 158
normal 158
reverse tick 180, 181
saddle-shaped 172–3
in ventricular hypertrophy 138, 139, 140
ST segment elevation acute coronary syndrome (STEACS) 159–69, 180
anterior 164, 180
inferior 165–6
lateral 165
localization 163–5

ST segment elevation myocardial
    infarction (STEMI) 160, 179,
    196–7
  reciprocal changes 177, 180
statins 168, 177
strain 139–40, 177, 182–3, 194,
    197–8
string galvanometer 270
stroke 44
subarachnoid haemorrhage 194
sudden cardiac death 57, 176, 204,
    209
supraventricular arrhythmia 243
supraventricular rhythm 69, 70
  with aberrant conduction 70–1,
    74–8
supraventricular tachycardia 24–5,
    59
  with aberrant conduction 265
  and bundle branch block 152
  distinction from ventricular
    tachycardia 71, 74–8
Swan–Ganz catheter 168
sweating 161
symptom diaries 234
syncope (fainting) 23, 25, 37, 51, 54,
    94–5, 125, 176, 225, 229, 230,
    237

T₃ 192, 216
T₄ 192, 216
T wave 2, 62, 186–200, 269
  and the axis 92
  definition 15, 18
  inversion 128–9, 139–41, 160–1,
    171, 173, 175, 177, 181–3,
    186–7, 193–9, 210, 214, 244
  in left bundle branch block 175
  in left ventricular hypertrophy
    138, 139
  normal 186–7, 193
  overlapping P waves 104
  in pericardial effusion 145
  pseudonormalization 177, 195
  and the QT interval 201–2
  in right ventricular hypertrophy
    139, 140
  small 190–2, 215

tall 141, 179, 187–90
tall, hyperacute 160, 161, 164,
    171, 188, 190
tented 188
and U waves 213–14
tachycardia 21, 24–7, 67, 210, 263
  atrial 24, 33–4, 36–9, 77, 181, 264
  AV junctional 103–4, 107
  AV nodal re-entry 33, 48–51, 72,
    77, 265
  AV re-entry 24, 30, 46–52, 77,
    114, 261, 265
  broad-complex 25, 53, 75–8, 258,
    259, 265
  and hyperthyroidism 216
  irregular narrow 264
  management 25–6, 222, 264–5
  narrow-complex 24, 258, 264–5
  and pacing 224
  paroxysmal 22, 36, 37, 117
  peri-arrest 264–5
  in pericardial tamponade 145
  in pulmonary embolism 129
  pulseless ventricular 255–7, 259,
    261
  regular narrow 265
  right ventricular outflow tract 55,
    64
  supraventricular 24–5, 59, 71,
    74–8, 152, 265
  ventricular 25
  see also sinus tachycardia;
    supraventricular tachycardia;
    ventricular tachycardia
tachycardia–bradycardia
    (tachy–brady) syndrome 22,
    36–7
tangent 90–1
tension pneumothorax 257
terfenadine 209
Thompson siphon recorder 269
thromboembolism 240, 257
  and atrial fibrillation 42, 43, 44, 45
  cerebral 40
thrombolysis 152, 161, 167–8, 225
thrombus 170
thyroid disorder 32–3, 41, 43, 190,
    192, 214, 216

thyroid-stimulating hormone 192, 216
thyrotoxicosis 206
torsades de pointes (polymorphic ventricular tachycardia) 25, 55, 56–7, 209, 211, 265
tracheal intubation 254
trauma 173, 207
treatment assessment 239
triangles, right-angled 89, 90–1
tricuspid stenosis 109
trifascicular block 95, 225
troponin I 162–3
troponin T 162–3
Trousseau's sign 208

U wave 2, 213–16
  definition 15, 16, 18
  and exercise ECG testing 240
  normal 213–14
  prominent 191, 205, 214–16
  and the QT interval 201–2
unconscious patients 66
  see also syncope
uraemia 32, 173
urea levels 206, 267
urine output 267

Valsalva manoeuvre 51, 52, 265
valve disease 44
vascular disease 44
vector analysis 89–92
vector diagrams 90
ventilation 254, 266
ventricle 10–13, 65
  accessory pathways 114–15
  and AV re-entry tachycardias 46
  dysfunction 241
  left 11–12
  pacemakers 227
  right 11–12, 165, 167
ventricular activity
  and atrial activity 72–4
  see also ventricular depolarization; ventricular repolarization
ventricular arrhythmia 25, 184, 211–12, 230, 243
ventricular bigeminy 62, 63, 68, 181

ventricular depolarization 11–13, 15, 18, 19, 69–70, 72–3
  and accessory pathways 114–15
  and the axis 84–5, 92
  and bundle branch block 147–51
  and myocardial infarction 132
  and the PR interval 113
  and the QRS complex 142–3, 147
ventricular ectopics 61–4, 68–70, 107, 153, 181
ventricular escape pacemaker 60
ventricular escape rhythm 22
ventricular fibrillation 25, 54, 57–8, 74, 209, 211
  diagnosis 258, 259
  fine 261
  inducible 204
  management 55, 230, 255–9, 261
  primary 57
  pulseless 258
  recurrent 58
  secondary 58
  and ventricular tachycardia 53
ventricular hypertrophy
  left 92, 109, 129, 133, 136–9
    and bundle branch block 152
    causes 139
    diagnostic criteria 137
    and ST segment depression 182
    and the T wave 197
  right 96, 97, 136, 139–40
    causes 139, 140
    and ST segment depression 182
    and the T wave 197
  with strain 139–40, 177, 182–3, 194, 197–8
ventricular pacemaker 31, 60
ventricular rate 19, 263
  assessment 67
  in atrial flutter 39
  control 45–6
  in ventricular tachycardia 53
ventricular repolarization 15, 18
  abnormally rapid 205
  axis for 92
  prolonged 211
  and the T wave 186

ventricular rhythm 30, 53–8, 146, 152–3
  assessment 65–71
  irregular 42–3, 67–9
  regular 67–9
ventricular tachycardia 25, 53–5, 70–1, 74, 211, 265
  and bundle branch block 152
  causes 54
  and digoxin toxicity 181
  distinction from supraventricular tachycardia 71, 74–8
  and exercise ECG testing 243
  with a focus in the left ventricle apex 96
  idiopathic 54, 55
  and left axis deviation 92, 96
  management 54–5, 230
  misdiagnosis 50
  non-sustained 243
  P waves in 105, 107
  polymorphic see torsades de pointes
  pulseless 255–7, 259, 261
  recurrent 55
  variants 56–7
verapamil 38–9
  in atrial fibrillation 43
  in atrial flutter 40
  in AV re-entry tachycardia 51–2
  drug interactions 39, 44, 52
vital signs 266
vitamin D 206, 208
vomiting 161
von Köllicker, Rudolph 268

Waller, Alexander D 269, 271
warfarin 44
waves
  history of 271
  nomenclature 2, 271
  size 2–3
  source 9–16
  see also specific waves
Wilson, Frank 271
Wolff–Parkinson–White (WPW) syndrome 48, 49, 51, 52
  asymptomatic 116
  and axis deviations 92, 96, 98
  and PR interval 113, 114–16
  and Q waves 129, 134
  and QRS abnormalities 153, 155–6
  and R waves 136, 140, 142
  and S waves 136, 142

x-ray see chest radiography

zero point (cardiac axis) 82